Core Principles of Adult Emergency Medicine

I0465445

Dr. Gregory C. Jackson
Dr. Victor S. Steller
Dr. Anthony S. Sasaki.
Dr. Peter C. Bryant

Preface

Emergency medicine is a dynamic and fast-paced field, requiring clinicians to possess a robust foundation of knowledge and the ability to make critical decisions under pressure. Core Principles of Adult Emergency Medicine is meticulously crafted to serve as a comprehensive guide for healthcare providers, bridging the gap between theoretical knowledge and practical application in emergency care.

This book was born from the collective expertise of four distinguished authors, each bringing a wealth of experience and diverse perspectives to the field. Dr. Gregory C. Jackson, Dr. Victor S. Steller, Dr. Anthony S. Sasaki, and Dr. Peter C. Bryant have collaborated to create an invaluable resource that emphasizes clarity, precision, and relevance to real-world scenarios. Their shared vision is to empower emergency care providers with the tools and confidence necessary to manage a wide spectrum of adult emergencies effectively.

Scope and Highlights

The content of this book spans a wide range of topics, carefully structured to address the key principles and challenges of adult emergency medicine:

1. Foundational Knowledge

The initial chapters establish a solid foundation by exploring the pathophysiology and epidemiology of common emergencies. These sections ensure a thorough understanding of the mechanisms underlying critical conditions.

2. Clinical Assessment and Decision-Making

Emphasis is placed on the systematic approach to patient evaluation, prioritizing swift yet accurate assessment methods. From recognizing subtle clinical signs to employing advanced diagnostic techniques, this book guides readers through the decision-making process in high-stakes environments.

3. **Evidence-Based Management**

Each chapter integrates the latest evidence-based guidelines and practices, ensuring readers have access to current and effective management strategies. Detailed discussions on pharmacological interventions, procedural techniques, and resuscitation protocols are presented clearly and concisely.

4. **Specialized Emergencies**

Specific focus is given to managing complex conditions such as cardiovascular crises, neurological emergencies, sepsis, and trauma. These chapters are augmented with case studies and algorithms to enhance comprehension and applicability.

5. **Ethical and Professional Considerations**

Beyond clinical skills, the book addresses the ethical dilemmas and communication challenges that are inherent to emergency medicine. These insights provide a holistic approach to patient care, fostering professionalism and empathy.

6. Future Directions and Innovations

Recognizing the evolving nature of emergency medicine, the book concludes with a forward-looking perspective, discussing emerging technologies, trends, and practices that are shaping the future of the field.

Target Audience

Core Principles of Adult Emergency Medicine is designed for a wide spectrum of readers, including medical students, residents, seasoned emergency medicine practitioners, and healthcare providers in related disciplines. Whether used as a reference guide or a learning tool, this book equips its audience with the essential knowledge and skills to excel in the demanding world of emergency medicine.

Acknowledgments

We extend our gratitude to the countless healthcare professionals who dedicate their lives to the field of emergency medicine. Their relentless commitment to patient care has been a constant source of inspiration. Special thanks also go to the research teams, editors, and contributors whose efforts have made this book possible.

It is our hope that this work will serve as a trusted companion in the journey of mastering adult emergency medicine, guiding clinicians to provide the highest standard of care in the moments when it matters most.

Dr. Gregory C. Jackson

Dr. Victor S. Steller

Dr. Anthony S. Sasaki

Dr. Peter C. Bryant

Preface

Acknowledgement

Table of contents

List of Abbreviations

Glossary

Table of contents

2. Essentials of Basic Life Support
- Activation of the Chain of Survival
- Dispatcher Assistance in BLS
- High-Quality Chest Compressions
- Role of Defibrillation in BLS

3. Chain of Survival
- Key Steps in the Chain
- Impact on Survival Rates
- Importance of Timely Interventions

4. Development of BLS Protocols
- Evidence-Based Guidelines
- Role of International Committees (ILCOR, AHA, ERC)

5. The DRSABCD Approach
- Steps in the Protocol
- Importance of Systematic Assessment

6. Adult BLS Sequence
- CAB vs. ABC Approach
- Regional Variations

7. Airway and Breathing Assessment
- Techniques for Airway Clearance

14. Rhythm Recognition in Cardiac Arrest
- Ventricular Fibrillation (VF)
- Pulseless Ventricular Tachycardia (VT)
- Asystole and Pulseless Electrical Activity (PEA)

15. Defibrillation Overview
- Pad Placement and Waveforms
- Energy Levels and Transthoracic Impedance Optimization

16. Concluding Remarks
- Importance of Continuous Training
- Future Directions in BLS Practices

Chapter 2: Critical Care Management – Focused Overview with Detailed Airway and Ventilation Protocols

1. Introduction to Critical Care Airway Management
- Importance of airway and ventilation in critical care
- Goals of airway management

2. Airway Management Techniques

- Initial airway assessment
- Clearing obstructions: Tools and methods
- Oxygen support and delivery methods

3. Breathing Evaluation and Oxygenation
- Assessment techniques and monitoring
- Non-Invasive Ventilation (NIV) approaches
- Role of BiPAP in respiratory failure

4. Rapid Sequence Intubation (RSI)
- Indications for RSI
- Pre-procedure preparation: Checklist and protocols
- Step-by-step RSI technique

5. Advanced Airway Management
- Managing difficult airways: Plan B strategies
- Verification of endotracheal tube placement
- Delayed Sequence Intubation (DSI)

6. Ventilation Strategies

- Protective ventilation for acute lung injury
- Apneic oxygenation techniques
- Controlled face mask ventilation

7. Airway Pharmacology
- Sedative agents
- Paralytic agents

8. Techniques to Improve Laryngoscopic View
- Positioning and maneuvers for optimal visualization
- Documentation of laryngoscopic grades

9. Confirmation of Endotracheal Tube Placement
- Role of capnography and colorimetric CO_2 detectors
- Adjunct methods

10. Complications of RSI and Management
- Common complications
- Strategies to address and mitigate risks

11. Face Mask Ventilation (FMV)
- Best practices for effective FMV
- Two-person techniques and adjuncts

12. Monitoring and Team Preparation
- Essential monitoring protocols during RSI
- Structured team and equipment readiness

Chapter 3: Oxygen Therapy – Table of Contents

1. Introduction to Oxygen Therapy
- Historical Perspective
- Importance of Oxygen in Cellular Function and Hypoxia Management

2. Uses of Supplemental Oxygen
- Airway Clearance Enhancement
- Pulmonary Gas Exchange Optimization
- Arterial Oxygen Saturation Improvement
- Increased Oxygen Demand Support
- Special Cases

3. Physiology of Oxygen Transport
- Ventilation Process and Pulmonary Gas Exchange
- Oxygen Binding and Transport in Blood

- Tissue Perfusion and Utilization
4. Ventilation and Hypoxia
   - Hypoxia Causes and Effects
   - Alveolar Gas Equation
5. Pulmonary Gas Exchange
   - Mechanisms and Efficiency Indicators
   - Impacts of Diffusion Impairments
6. Oxygen Carriage in the Blood
   - Hemoglobin's Role and Dissociation Curve Analysis
   - Factors Influencing Oxygen Release
7. Oxygen Flux and Delivery
   - Calculation and Clinical Implications
   - Challenges in Illness or Injury
8. Tissue Oxygenation
   - Local Perfusion and Diffusion Dynamics
   - Increased Demand Scenarios
9. Oxygen Delivery Systems
   - Overview
   - Fixed-Performance Systems:

- Variable-Performance Systems:

10. One Hundred Percent Oxygen Delivery Systems
    - Free-Flowing Circuits
    - Reservoir Systems
    - Demand Valve Systems
    - Closed-Circuit Systems

11. Manual Ventilation Systems
    - Advantages and Limitations

12. Helium and Oxygen Mixtures (Heliox)
    - Mechanism of Action and Clinical Applications
    - Benefits and Constraints

13. Oxygen Therapy in Clinical Practice
    - Introduction to Oxygen Therapy
    - Importance of Oxygen in Clinical Settings
    - Indications for Oxygen Therapy

13. Measurement of Oxygenation
    - Clinical Assessment and Limitations
    - Arterial Blood Gasses (ABG) and Pulse Oximetry

- Factors Affecting Pulse
  Oximetry Accuracy

14. Oxygen Therapy in
Pediatric Patients

- Physiological and
  Anatomical
  Considerations
- Equipment and
  Techniques for Pediatric
  Oxygen Delivery
- Managing Psychological
  Challenges
- Risks of Oxygen
  Toxicity in Infants and
  Children

15. Oxygen Therapy During
Patient Transfer

- Role of Supplemental
  Oxygen in Transport
- Equipment and
  Monitoring
  Requirements
- Challenges in Air Travel

16. Oxygen Therapy for
Specific Conditions

- Asthma
- Managing Hypoxia and
  Ventilation Strategies
- Chronic Obstructive
  Pulmonary Disease
  (COPD)
- Oxygen Titration and
  Blood Gas Monitoring

- Management of Hypercapnia and Ventilatory Failure

17. Specialized Oxygen Delivery Techniques
- High-Flow Oxygen Therapy and Humidification
- Continuous Positive Airway Pressure (CPAP)
- Non-Invasive Positive-Pressure Ventilation (NIPPV)

18. Hyperbaric Oxygen Therapy (HBO)
- Indications and Mechanisms
- Benefits for Carbon Monoxide Poisoning and Ischemic Conditions

19. Complications and Risks of Oxygen Therapy
- Equipment-Related Issues
- Carbon Dioxide Narcosis
- Oxygen Toxicity and Free Radical Damage

20. Recent Advances and Research in Oxygen Therapy
- Titrated Oxygen Therapy in Acute and Chronic Conditions

- Emerging Evidence for Safety and Efficacy

Chapter 4: Haemodynamic Monitoring in the Emergency Department

1. Introduction to Haemodynamic Monitoring
   - Importance in Emergency Care
   - Historical Evolution
2. Practical Considerations
   - Basic vs. Advanced Monitoring Techniques
   - Clinical Relevance and Decision-Making
   - Risks and Limitations
3. Key Principles for Effective Monitoring
   - Clinical Utility and Simplicity
   - Accuracy, Continuity, and Safety
4. Cardiovascular Physiology
   - Understanding Cardiac Output and Cardiac Index
   - Factors Influencing Haemodynamics
5. Non-Invasive Monitoring Techniques
   - Blood Pressure Measurement

- Historical Methods and Modern Devices
- Automated Oscillometric Systems
- Ultrasonic Cardiac Output Monitoring (USCOM)
- Oesophageal Doppler
- Transthoracic Echocardiography

6. Invasive Monitoring Techniques
- Arterial Blood Pressure Monitoring
- Procedure and Applications
- Central Venous Pressure Monitoring
- Central Venous Access: Indications and Complications
- Central Venous Oxygen Saturation

7. Advanced Monitoring Technologies
- Transpulmonary Thermodilution
- Parameters: ITBV, EVLW, and CFI
- PiCCO System Overview
- Advantages and Limitations

8. Applications in Emergency Department Scenarios
- Sepsis Management and Goal-Directed Therapy
- Haemodynamic Assessment in Heart Failure and Shock

9. Future Directions
- Emerging Technologies
- Evidence-Based Advancements in ED Monitoring

Chapter 5: Shock Overview

1. Introduction to Shock
- Definition and Clinical Significance
- Early vs. Late-Stage Shock
- Challenges in Recognition
- Classification of Shock

2. Aetiology and Epidemiology
- Contributing Factors
- Physiological Classifications
- Pathophysiology of Shock
- Mechanisms of Perfusion Failure
- Compensatory Mechanisms
- Progression to Decompensated Shock

3. Clinical Features
- Mental State Alterations
- Circulatory and Skin Changes
- Hemodynamic Parameters
- Organ Dysfunction

4. Initial Management of Shock
- Structured Protocols (ATLS, ACLS)
- Role of Multidisciplinary Teams
- Urgent Interventions
- Advanced Diagnostic Tools
- Role of Echocardiography and Ultrasound
- Invasive Monitoring Techniques

5. Goal-Directed Resuscitation
- Evidence-Based Practices
- Customizing Goals to Patient Needs

6. Fluid Therapy in Shock Management
- Fluid Selection and Administration
- Routes of Administration
- Complications of Fluid Therapy

7. Use of Inotropes and Vasopressors
- Mechanisms of Action
- Drug Selection and Administration
- Titration and Monitoring

8. Absolute Hypovolemia
- Clinical Features and Investigations
- Imaging and Surgical Interventions

9. Complications and Common Pitfalls in Shock Management
- Delayed Diagnosis
- Inadequate Resuscitation
- Mismanagement of Therapy

10. Future Directions in Shock Management
- Emerging Technologies
- Personalized Treatment Approaches

11. Comprehensive Management of Shock Syndromes
- Introduction to Shock Syndromes
- Definition and Classification of Shock
- Diagnostic Approaches
- Hypovolemic Shock
- Cardiogenic Shock
- Obstructive Shock

- Cardiac Tamponade: Diagnosis and Management
- Pulmonary Embolism: Identification and Intervention
- Tension Pneumothorax: Clinical Signs and Emergency Treatment

12. Distributive Shock
- Septic Shock
- Epidemiology and Pathogenesis
- Screening and Diagnostic Criteria
- Management: Antibiotics, Fluid Resuscitation, and Vasopressors
- Neurogenic Shock
- Etiology: Acute Spinal Cord Injury
- Clinical Features and Supportive Treatment
- Anaphylactic Shock
- Pathophysiology and Trigger Identification
- Emergency Management: Epinephrine and Adjunct Therapies

13. Adrenal Shock

- Quality Improvement Initiatives

17. Case Studies and Clinical Scenarios
    - Real-World Applications of Shock Management Principles
    - Lessons Learned and Pitfalls to Avoid

18. Summary and Future Directions
    - Key Takeaways
    - Ongoing Research and Innovations in Shock Management

Chapter 6: Arterial Blood Gasses (ABG)

1. Introduction to Arterial Blood Gas (ABG) Analysis
    - Overview of ABG's role in emergency medicine
    - Importance of accurate interpretation for patient management

2. Technical Aspects of Arterial Blood Gas Analysis
    - History and development of ABG electrodes
    - Role of the Clarke and Severinghaus electrodes
    - Co-oximetry and blood gas analyzers

3. Collection and Handling of Blood Samples
- Guidelines for proper sample collection
- Importance of sample transport and temperature stabilization

4. Arterial Puncture Technique
- Common sites for blood collection
- The Modified Allen test and its role

5. Indwelling Arterial Catheters
- Indications for continuous monitoring
- Aseptic techniques and potential complications

6. Interpretation of ABG Results
- Gas Exchange and Respiratory Failure
- Hypoxemia and hypercapnia
- Type I and Type II respiratory failure
- Alveolar–Arterial Oxygen Gradient
- Calculation and clinical significance
- Oxygen Delivery and Hemoglobin Saturation
- Oxygen content and its clinical relevance

- Oxygen-Hemoglobin Dissociation Curve
- Influence of PaCO2, pH, and temperature on oxygen delivery

7. Pathophysiology of Hypoxemic Respiratory Failure
- Mechanisms of hypoxemia and treatment approaches

8. Neurological Complications and Treatment Approaches Post-Cardiac Arrest
- High Incidence of Neurological Injury
- Impact of reperfusion injury and biochemical processes
- Uncertainty in Physiological Targets
- Oxygen, CO2, blood pressure, and temperature management
- Current limitations and treatment gaps

9. Pathophysiology of Cerebral Ischemia and Reperfusion Injury
- Cellular mechanisms of ischemic injury and post-ROSC effects

10. Cerebral Hemodynamics Post-Reperfusion

Chapter 7: Anaphylaxis
A Comprehensive Guide for
Medical Practitioners
1. Introduction

- Definition and Overview of Anaphylaxis
- Historical Context and Terminology

2. Classification of Anaphylaxis
   - Overview of International Definitions
   - NIAID/FAAN Criteria
   - Grading Systems

3. Etiology and Risk Factors
   - Common Triggers of Anaphylaxis
   - Risk Factors and Summation Anaphylaxis
   - Geographical Variation in Triggers

4. Pathophysiology
   - Immune-Mediated (IgE and IgG4) Mechanisms
   - Non-IgE-Mediated Anaphylaxis
   - Cellular Activation and Mediator Release
   - Modulation and Pharmacological Effects of Mediators

5. Clinical Manifestations
   - Cutaneous Symptoms
   - Respiratory and Systemic Symptoms

- Cardiovascular and Neurological Manifestations
- Gastrointestinal Symptoms

6. Differential Diagnosis
- Conditions with Similar Presentations
- Diagnostic Considerations

7. Clinical Investigations and Laboratory Assessment
- Diagnosis Based on Clinical Presentation
- Use of Diagnostic Tests

8. Anaphylaxis Management
- Immediate Management (Epinephrine, Oxygen, Fluids)
- Secondary Interventions (Antihistamines, Corticosteroids, etc.)
- Management of β-Blocked Patients (Glucagon, Atropine, Salbutamol)
- Role of Corticosteroids and Antihistamines in Treatment

9. Discharge and Long-Term Management
- Post-Recovery Monitoring

- Discharge Protocols
- Epinephrine Auto-Injector and Allergen Management Plan
- Referral to Allergists and Patient Education

10. Special Considerations
- Drug-Induced Anaphylaxis (Penicillin, NSAIDs, etc.)
- Insect Sting and Food-Induced Anaphylaxis
- Perioperative and Latex-Induced Anaphylaxis

11. Conclusion
- Key Takeaways
- Future Directions and Research Needs

Chapter 8 (A): Trauma

1. Epidemiology of Trauma
- Global impact and leading causes of trauma-related deaths
- Trauma-related mortality in high-income vs. developing countries
- Economic and social consequences

2. Advances in Trauma Systems
- Impact of prevention initiatives

- Historical development of trauma care systems
- The trimodal distribution of trauma deaths and interventions

3. Key Elements of a Trauma Care System
- Primary Objectives
- Initial Patient Management (ABCDE approach)
- Continuous Quality Improvement

4. The Trauma System: Pre-Hospital and In-Hospital Phases
- Pre-Hospital Care
- In-Hospital Trauma Response

5. Essential Management Phases in Trauma Care
- Airway Management
- Breathing and Ventilation
- Shock Management

6. Disability and Neurological Assessment
- Glasgow Coma Scale and neurological evaluation
- Imaging for suspected head injuries

7. Exposure and Temperature Control
- Managing hypothermia in trauma patients
- The debate over therapeutic hypothermia for head injuries

8. Next Steps and Specialized Care
- Coordination of care and involvement of specialists
- Imaging and secondary surveys

9. Quality Improvement in Trauma Care
- Trauma Quality Improvement (TQI) programs
- Importance of trauma registries for outcomes assessment

10. Trauma in Developing Countries
- Trauma burden and public health initiatives
- Implementation of trauma systems and education programs

11. Neurotrauma
- Overview and prevalence of neurotrauma in trauma patients

- Pathogenesis of primary and secondary brain injuries
- Classification of primary neurotrauma injuries
- Skull Fractures
- Concussion and Second Impact Syndrome
- Contusion and Intracranial Hematomas
- Diffuse Axonal Injury (DAI)
- Penetrating Injury

Table of Contents: Chapter 8(B) – Spinal Trauma

1. Essentials
- Clinical Examination and Criteria for Spinal Injuries
- Importance of Early Detection and Secondary Injury Prevention
- Spinal Immobilization and Complications
- Use of Methylprednisolone in SCI Management

2. Overview of Spinal Cord Injury (SCI)
- Primary Causes and Risk Factors in SCI
- Preventable Neurological Deterioration in SCI

- Impacts on Patients and Communities

3. Pathophysiology
   - Levels of Vertebral Injury
   - Associated Injuries and Secondary Trauma
   - Effects of Spinal Cord Injury on the Autonomic Nervous System

4. Pre-Hospital Management
   - Extrication and Immobilization Techniques
   - In-line Spinal Protection
   - Initial Treatment and Primary Survey

5. Mechanisms of Spinal Injuries
   - Flexion-Rotation
   - Vertebral Compression
   - Lateral Flexion
   - Distraction

6. Cervical Spine Injuries
   - C1 (Atlas) Fractures
   - C2 (Axis) Fractures
   - C3–C7 Fractures

7. Thoracic and Thoracolumbar Spine Injuries
   - Thoracic Spine Injuries
   - Thoracolumbar Spine Injuries

8. Lumbar Spine Injuries

- Seatbelt and Hyperflexion Injuries

9. Imaging and Diagnosis
   - Plain Films: Initial Imaging Techniques
   - Advanced Imaging: CT and MRI
   - Specific Radiological Findings for Spinal Injuries

10. Specific Fractures
    - Chance Fractures
    - Burst and Compression Fractures

Chapter 8 (C): Facial Trauma Assessment and Management in the Emergency Department (ED)

1. Prevalence and Causes of Facial Injuries
   - Demographics and Risk Factors
   - Common Causes of Facial Trauma
   - Trends in Developed vs. Developing Countries

2. Anatomy and Functions of the Face
   - Bony Structure and Soft Tissue Support
   - Key Organs and Functions

- Importance of Facial Appearance and Function in Trauma Care
3. Associated Injuries
    - High-Energy vs. Low-Energy Trauma
    - Age-Related Considerations in Trauma
4. History and Primary Survey
    - Mechanism of Injury and Risk Stratification
    - Considerations for Intimate Partner Violence
    - Primary Survey Protocol
5. Airway Management
    - Challenges in Airway Management with Facial Trauma
    - Techniques for Airway Stabilization
    - Surgical Considerations for Severe Trauma
6. Breathing and Circulation
    - Assessing Respiratory Function in Facial Trauma
    - Hemorrhage Control and Management Strategies
    - Special Considerations for Nasal and Pharyngeal Packing

1. Soft Tissue Injuries
- Lacerations, Abrasions, and Burns
- Principles of Wound Care and Repair
2. Facial Fractures
- Mandibular, Zygomatic, and Orbital FracturesLe Fort and Nasal Fractures
- Diagnosis and Surgical Management
3. Penetrating Facial Injuries
- Gunshot Wounds, Stabbings, and Impaling Objects
- Airway Management in Penetrating Trauma

Chapter 8 (D): Abdominal Trauma

1. Introduction to Abdominal Trauma
- Overview of abdominal injuries in trauma
- Importance of early diagnosis and high suspicion
- Goals of initial care and involvement of trauma surgeons

2. Primary and Secondary Surveys

- Primary survey and identification of potential hemorrhage
- Comprehensive abdominal examination
- Secondary survey and focused examination areas

3. History Taking
   - Mechanism of injury and its role in diagnosis
   - The AMPLE acronym for trauma history

4. Abdominal Examination
   - Clinical signs of penetrating vs. blunt trauma
   - Specific injury patterns and physical findings
   - Back, rectal, and vaginal examinations in trauma cases

5. Key Risk Factors for Abdominal Injury
   - Risk factors including vehicle collisions, falls, and hypotension

6. Essentials for Diagnosis and Management
   - Importance of early detection
   - Role of CT and FAST in diagnosis

- Need for senior trauma surgeon involvement

7. Investigations
   - Initial trauma workup: Blood tests and imaging
   - Limitations of abdominal radiography
   - Role of laparotomy for gunshot or stab wounds

8. Abdominal CT vs. Ultrasound
   - CT imaging: Benefits and limitations
   - Ultrasound: Bedside tool for unstable patients

9. Interventional Radiology
   - Increasing role in managing retroperitoneal and pelvic bleeding
   - Hybrid suites for streamlined care

10. Focused Assessment with Sonography in Trauma (FAST)
    - Role of FAST in abdominal trauma diagnosis
    - Sensitivity, specificity, and limitations of FAST

Chapter 8 (E): Chest Trauma

1. Introduction
   - Incidence of thoracic trauma

- Blunt trauma statistics and regional variations

2. Principles of Initial Management
   - Oxygenation and ventilatory support
   - Pleural and pericardial decompression
   - Circulatory support and pain management
   - Imaging protocols and life-threatening injury identification

3. Oxygenation
   - Supplemental oxygen strategies
   - Advanced techniques for severe hypoxia

5. Pulmonary Support
   - Pain management and its impact on ventilation
   - Non-invasive vs. mechanical ventilation

6. Fluid Resuscitation
   - Permissive hypotension in penetrating trauma
   - Fluid management in blunt trauma and pulmonary contusion

7. Analgesia
   - Pain management strategies for rib

fractures and chest
trauma

8. Indications for Emergency
Thoracotomy
- Cardiac tamponade,
thoracic vascular
injuries, and other
surgical indications
- Importance of timely
intervention

9. Thoracic Injuries
- Fractured ribs and
associated complications
- Sternal fractures and
myocardial contusion
- Vertebral and spinal cord
injuries
- Flail chest management

10. Myocardial Laceration and
Cardiac Tamponade
- Diagnosis and
management strategies
- Role of bedside
sonography

11. Tension
Pneumopericardium
- Pathophysiology,
diagnosis, and urgent
management

12. Thoracic Aortic Transection
- Mechanisms, diagnosis,
and treatment strategies

- Importance of early intervention and imaging

13. Esophageal Perforation
- Diagnosis and management of blunt trauma-related esophageal rupture

14. Future Considerations
- Emerging technologies in diagnosis and treatment
- Advances in imaging, non-invasive ventilation, and rib fixation

Chapter 8 (F)
Limb Trauma

1. Introduction
- Overview of Limb Injuries
- Scope and Clinical Significance
- Holistic Approach in Trauma Care

2. Primary and Secondary Surveys
- Primary Survey Prioritization
- Addressing Circulatory Complications
- Secondary Survey and Orthopedic Assessment

3. Types of Fractures
- Classification of Fractures

- Management of Closed vs. Open Fractures
- High-Risk Fractures and Associated Complications

4. Associated Injuries
   - Vascular Injury
   - Recognition and Diagnostic Tools
   - Sites and Types of Arterial Damage
   - Nerve Injury
   - Mechanisms and Classification
   - Clinical Presentations and Treatment

5. Clinical Assessment and Diagnosis
   - History Taking and MIST Framework
   - Physical Examination
   - Inspection and Palpation
   - Vascular and Neurological Assessments

6. Splinting in Limb Trauma
   - Principles and Benefits
   - Types of Splints
   - Complications and Precautions

7. Definitive Management

- Principles of Effective Wound Irrigation
- Appropriate Use of Antiseptics
- Techniques for Reducing Infection Risks

12. Managing the Mangled Extremity
- Prioritization of Life-Threatening Injuries
- Limb Alignment and Vascular Assessment
- Pain Management and Surgical Consultation

13. Hyperbaric Oxygen Therapy (HBOT)
- Indications and Controversies
- Applications in Crush Injuries and Compartment Syndrome

14. Disposition and Post-Trauma Care
- ED Stabilization and Follow-Up Plans
- Discharge Instructions for Cast and Splint Management
- Considerations for Elderly and High-Risk Patients

15. Surgical Intervention and Operating Theatre Procedures

- Indications for Urgent Surgical Management
- Damage-Control Surgery Principles

16. Complications in Trauma Management
- Identification and Treatment of Compartment Syndrome
- Monitoring and Interventions for Acute Limb Ischemia

17. Immobilization and Its Consequences
- Risks Associated with Prolonged Immobilization
- Prevention and Management of Complications

18. Radiation Hazards in Trauma Care
- ALARA Principle and Safe Imaging Practices
- Risks of Ionizing Radiation and Mitigation Strategies

19. Trauma Imaging Protocols
- Essential Initial Imaging Procedures
- Advanced Imaging Techniques for Complex Injuries

- History and Risk Factors
- Physical Examination
- Imaging and Investigations
- Principles of Wound Cleaning and Repair
- Cleaning Procedures and Techniques
- Debridement Methods
- Suture Selection and Timing

22. Tetanus Prophylaxis and Wound Healing
- Phases of Wound Healing
- Tetanus Immunization Protocols
- Healing by Secondary Intention

23. Suturing Techniques and Knot Management
- Needle and Suture Selection
- Basic Suture Techniques
- Approaches to Linear and Complex Wounds
- Edge Eversion and Wound Approximation
- Knot Tying: Methods and Precautions

24. Postoperative Care and Follow-Up

- Antibiotics and Infection Prevention
- Physical Therapy and Splinting
- Suture Removal and Handling

25. Special Considerations
- Managing Wounds with Embedded Foreign Bodies
- Wounds in High-Risk Populations
- Referral Guidelines for Complex Wounds

Chapter 8 (G): Burns

1. Introduction to Burn Care
- Advances in Burn Management
- Burn-Related Mortality and Risk Factors

2. Pathophysiology of Burns
- Structure and Functions of the Skin
- Zones of Injury in Burns
- Classification of Burns
- Depth of Burns
- Epidermal Burns

3. Partial-Thickness Burns (Superficial, Mid-Dermal, Deep)
- Full-Thickness Burns
- Burn Etiology: Thermal, Chemical, and Electrical

4. Assessment and Evaluation
- History and Initial Examination
- Rule of Nines and Lund-Browder Chart
- Recognizing Inhalation Injuries

5. Burn Management
- Pre-Hospital Management
- Emergency Department Care
- Airway Management
- Pain Management
- Prevention of Hypothermia
- Fluid Resuscitation Protocols

6. Subsequent Care for Burn Patients
- Wound Care and Debridement
- Skin Grafting and Escharotomy
- Facial and Eye Burn Management
- Tetanus Prophylaxis

7. Complications of Burns
- Burn Shock
- Infection and Sepsis
- Coagulation Dysfunction

8. Inhalation Injuries

- Pathophysiology of Smoke Inhalation
- Carbon Monoxide and Cyanide Toxicity
- Pulmonary Complications

9. Chemical Burns
- Mechanisms of Injury (Coagulation vs. Liquefaction Necrosis)
- Decontamination and Irrigation Protocols
- Special Considerations for Alkali and Acid Burns

10. Disposition and Burn Unit Transfer
- Criteria for Burn Center Referral
- Transportation and Stabilization

11. Massive Transfusion in Burn Care
- Definition and Activation Protocols
- Fresh Frozen Plasma and Platelet Transfusion Guidelines
- Role of Cryoprecipitate and Calcium Administration
- Use of Synthetic Agents

12. Future Directions in Burn Management
- Emerging Technologies in Burn Wound Healing
- Advances in Inhalation Injury Treatment

Chapter 9 (A): Orthopedic Emergencies

1. Introduction to Orthopedic Emergencies
- Overview and Scope

2. Clavicle Fractures
- Epidemiology and Anatomy
- Mechanism of Injury and Clinical Presentation
- Diagnosis and Imaging
- Non-Surgical Management
- Surgical Management and Indications
- Complications and Outcomes

3. Acromioclavicular Joint (AC) Injuries
- Mechanism of Injury
- Tossy-Rockwood Classification
- Diagnostic Approach
- Management Based on Severity

4. Sternoclavicular Joint Dislocation

- Anterior vs. Posterior Dislocation
- Risk of Neurovascular Injury
- Diagnosis and Imaging Modalities
- Management and Reduction Techniques

5. Scapular Fractures
- Epidemiology and Associated Injuries
- Classification and Clinical Evaluation
- Conservative vs. Surgical Management
- Floating Shoulder: Special Considerations

6. Supraspinatus Tendon Injuries
- Pathophysiology and Clinical Signs
- Diagnostic Tests
- Treatment Strategies

7. Shoulder Dislocations
- Types: Anterior, Posterior, Inferior (Luxatio Erecta)
- Mechanism of Injury and Neurovascular Assessment
- Management Approaches
- Non-Surgical Reduction Techniques:

- FARES Technique
- Spaso Technique
- Modified Kocher Maneuver
- Scapular Manipulation
- Posterior and Inferior Dislocations: Special Considerations

8. Post-Reduction Care
- Rehabilitation and Pain Management
- Monitoring for Recurrence or Complications

9. Surgical Management in Specific Cases
- Indications for Surgical Intervention
- Long-Term Outcomes and Prognosis

Chapter 9 (B): Elbow Dislocations – A Detailed Analysis and Approach

1. Introduction to Elbow Dislocations
- Prevalence and Clinical Significance
- Anatomy and Stability of the Elbow Joint

2. Classification of Elbow Dislocations
- Posterior Dislocations

- Postero-Medial and Postero-Lateral Types
- Anterior Dislocations
- Anteromedial and Anterolateral Types
- Special Cases:
- Monteggia Fracture
- The "Terrible Triad" of the Elbow

3. Clinical Evaluation
- History and Physical Examination
- Identification of Neurovascular Complications
- Differentiating Dislocations from Complex Fractures

4. Diagnostic Imaging
- Standard Radiographic Views
- Role of Computed Tomography (CT)
- Duplex Doppler Ultrasound for Vascular Injury

5. Management Approach
- Reduction Techniques
- General Approach to Closed Reduction
- Special Considerations for Complex Dislocations

- Post-Reduction Stability Assessment
- Valgus, Varus, and Lateral Pivot-Shift Tests

6. Post-Reduction Care
- Radiographic Confirmation
- Immobilization and Splinting Guidelines
- Early Mobilization vs. Prolonged Immobilization

7. Surgical Considerations
- Indications for Surgical Intervention
- Techniques for Managing Fractures and Instability
- Outcomes of Surgical vs. Conservative Treatment

8. Ulnar Nerve Injuries in Elbow Dislocations
- Prevalence and Clinical Indicators
- Conservative vs. Surgical Management

9. Disposition and Follow-Up Care
- Emergency Department Discharge Criteria
- Early Mobilization Protocols

- Long-Term Functional Recovery

Chapter 9 (C): Fractures of the Proximal Humerus

1. Introduction
   - Overview of shoulder girdle functionality
   - Impact of humerus fractures on upper limb function
   - Categories of humerus fractures

2. Fractures of the Proximal Humerus
   - Injury Patterns
   - Prevalence and demographics
   - Common causes and mechanisms
   - Clinical Assessment
   - Presentation and physical examination
   - Neurovascular considerations
   - Evaluating underlying medical conditions

3. Diagnostic Imaging
   - Standard radiographic views
   - Advanced imaging modalities

4. Classification of Proximal Humerus Fractures

- Neer classification system
- One-part fractures
- Two-part fractures
- Three- and four-part fractures

5. Management and Treatment
- Conservative management
- Sling immobilization and pain control
- Prognosis for one- and two-part fractures
- Surgical intervention
- Open reduction and internal fixation (ORIF)
- Factors influencing surgical decisions
- Role of locking-plate technology

6. Special Considerations
- Fractures at the anatomical neck and articular surface
- Risk of avascular necrosis
- Indications for humeral hemiarthroplasty
- Fracture dislocations
- Associated injuries and reduction techniques

7. Disposition and Follow-Up

- Discharge criteria for non-displaced fractures
- Indications for orthopedic consultation
- Screening for osteoporosis in elderly patients

8. Fractures of the Humeral Shaft
- Injury Patterns
- Demographics and mechanisms
- Clinical Presentation
- Symptoms and associated injuries

9. Management of Humeral Shaft Fractures
- Non-surgical management
- Immobilization techniques and acceptable deformity criteria
- Surgical repair
- Indications and outcomes

10. Radial Nerve Injury in Humeral Shaft Fractures
- Prevalence and clinical features
- Management and prognosis

11. Distal Humerus Fractures

- Classification and injury mechanisms
- Clinical Assessment and Imaging
- Diagnostic techniques and imaging modalities
- Treatment and Management
- Non-surgical and surgical approaches

Chapter 9(D): Radial Head Fractures: Comprehensive Clinical Overview

1. Clinical Presentation
   - History
   - Examination
2. Diagnostic Investigations
   - Imaging
3. Classification of Radial Head Fractures
   - Type I: Displacement
   - Type II: Displacement
   - Type III: Comminuted Fracture
   - Type IV: Fracture with Elbow Dislocation
4. Management Approaches
   - Non-Operative Treatment
   - Surgical Options
   - Management of Radial Neck Fractures
   - Essex-Lopresti Fractures

5. Complications
- Neurovascular Injuries
- Movement Limitations

6. Essential Points for Emergency Management
- General Principles
- Specific Techniques for Related Injuries
- Colles Fracture
- Smith Fracture
- Barton Fracture
- Radial Styloid Fracture
- Ulnar Styloid Fracture
- Carpal Fractures and Dislocations
- Wrist Dislocations

7. Introduction to Hand Injuries in Emergency Care
- Epidemiology
- Impact on Daily Activities

8. Clinical Features of Hand Injuries
- History Taking
- Examination Procedures

9. Clinical Investigations
- Imaging Techniques
- Role of Ultrasound and MRI

10. Management of Common Hand Injuries
- Pain Management
- Wound Care

- Tendon and Ligament
  Injury Management
11. Fingertip Injuries
- Conservative Care
- Surgical Interventions for
  Severe Cases
12. Conclusion
- Summary of Key
  Management Principles
- Future Directions in
  Emergency Hand Care

Chapter 9 (E): Pelvic Injuries

1. Anatomy of the Pelvic Ring
- Components of the
  Pelvic Ring
- Ligamentous Integrity
  and Structural Support
2. Classification of Pelvic
Fractures
- Open vs. Closed
  Fractures
- Stable vs. Unstable
  Fractures
- Young and Resnik
  Classification
3. Types of Compression
Injuries
  1. Lateral Compression
     Injuries
- Type 1: Sacral
  Compression and Pubic
  Ramus Fractures

- Type 2: Iliac Wing Fractures and Sacroiliac Disruption
- Type 3: Combined Lateral and Anteroposterior Injuries
2. Anteroposterior Compression Injuries
- Type 1: Minimal Diastasis
- Type 2: Severe "Open-Book" Injuries
- Type 3: Complete Ligamentous Disruption
3. Vertical Shear Injuries (Malgaigne Fracture)

4. Clinical Assessment of Pelvic Fractures
- Primary Trauma Protocol
- Physical Examination
- Radiographic Assessment

5. Complications Associated with Pelvic Fractures
- Hemorrhage and Management Strategies
- Genitourinary and Bladder Injuries
- Urethral and Genital Injuries

6. Management of Unstable Pelvic Fractures

- Initial Stabilization and Splinting
- Advanced Surgical Interventions

7. Open Pelvic Fractures
- Characteristics and Risks
- Management Strategies

8. Acetabular Fractures
- Clinical Features
- Diagnostic Imaging
- Management

9. Stable Pelvic Fractures
- Isolated Pubic Ramus Fractures
- Iliac Wing Fractures (Duverney Fracture)
- Isolated Avulsion Fractures
- Anterior Superior Iliac Spine Fractures
- Anterior Inferior Iliac Spine Fractures
- Ischial Tuberosity Fractures
- Coccygeal Fractures

10. Management of Isolated Stable Fractures
- Conservative Treatment Approaches
- Gradual Mobilization and Recovery Strategies

Chapter 9 (F): Hip Joint Fractures – A Comprehensive Overview

1. Anatomy and Blood Supply of the Hip Joint
- Anatomy of the Hip Joint
- Blood Supply to the Hip
- Trochanteric Arterial Ring
- Retinacular Arteries and Avascular Necrosis (AVN)
2. Avascular Necrosis (AVN)
- Definition and Pathophysiology
- Radiographic Features
- Risk Reduction in Dislocations
3. Classification of Hip Fractures
- Intracapsular Fractures
- Femoral Head and Neck
- Garden Classification for Femoral Neck Fractures
- Extracapsular Fractures
- Intertrochanteric and Subtrochanteric Types
4. Management of Hip Fractures
- Intracapsular Fractures
- Treatment Options

- Complications: AVN, Non-union, and Post-Traumatic Arthritis
- Extracapsular Fractures
- Open Reduction and Internal Fixation (ORIF)
- Management of Associated Risks
5. Complications of Hip Fractures
- Mortality and Morbidity
- Specific Risks: Infection, Osteomyelitis, and AVN
6. Hip Dislocations
- Allis Maneuver and Other Relocation Techniques
- Complications of Delayed Reduction
7. Anterior Hip Dislocations
- Mechanism of Injury
- Classification: Superior and Inferior Dislocations
- Clinical Assessment and Neurovascular Examination
- Imaging and Diagnostic Tools
- Management and Long-Term Outcomes
8. Summary of Key Points

- Overview of Hip Fracture and Dislocation Management
- Importance of Early Diagnosis and Treatment
- Complications and Preventive Strategies

Chapter 9 (G): Femoral Shaft Fractures – Mechanism, Classification, and Management

1. Mechanism of Injury
- High-Energy Trauma
- Contributing Factors: Osteoporosis and Metastatic Bone Disease

2. Classification of Femoral Shaft Fractures
- Open vs. Closed Fractures
- Fracture Types: Transverse, Oblique, Spiral, and Segmental
- Fracture Location: Proximal, Midshaft, and Distal Third
- Associated Characteristics

3. Stress Fractures of the Femur
- Causes and Risk Factors
- Clinical Presentation
- Diagnostic Tools

- Conservative Treatment Approach

4. Clinical Assessment
   - Physical Examination Findings
   - Neurovascular Injury Evaluation

5. Vascular Injury in Femoral Shaft Fractures
   - Pathophysiology: Haematoma and Arterial Damage
   - Diagnostic Modalities: Doppler Imaging and Arteriography
   - Management of Vascular Compromise

6. Associated Injuries
   - Pelvic Fractures and Hip Dislocations
   - Knee Ligament and Meniscal Injuries
   - Blood Loss and Hemodynamic Considerations

7. Management of Femoral Shaft Fractures
   - Initial Priorities
   - Hemorrhage Control
   - Pain Management and Stabilization

- Role of Early Reduction and Radiographic Evaluation

Chapter 9 (H): Analgesia and Management of Fractures and Knee Injuries

1. Pain Management in Emergency Settings
   - Intravenous Opioid Analgesia
   - Role of Femoral Nerve Block
2. Fracture Reduction and Splinting
   - Principles of Immediate Reduction
   - Splint Types (Donway, Hare Traction Splints)
3. Fluid Resuscitation for Fractures
   - Estimating Blood Loss
   - Fluid and Blood Product Management
   - Monitoring with Indwelling Catheters
4. Orthopedic Intervention
   - Early Surgical Fixation (Intramedullary Nailing)
   - Management of Open Fractures
5. Complications of Femoral Fractures

- Immediate: Fat Embolism, Hemorrhagic Shock, ARDS
- Long-Term: Non-Union, Limb Shortening, Malalignment

6. Detailed Overview of Knee Anatomy
- Structural and Functional Aspects of the Knee Joint
- Role of Ligaments, Muscles, and Tendons in Stability

7. Clinical Examination of Knee Injuries
- History Taking: Mechanism and Nature of Injury
- Physical Examination: Inspection, Palpation, and Movement Tests
- Stability Tests (Drawer Tests, Lachman, McMurray, and Apley)

8. Radiographic and Imaging Studies
- X-rays: AP, Lateral, and Specialized Views
- CT and MRI for Fracture and Soft-Tissue Assessment

9. Types of Fractures
- Distal Femur Fractures

- Tibial Plateau Fractures and Schatzker Classification

10. Knee Dislocations
    - Tibiofemoral Dislocation: Assessment and Management
    - Patellar Dislocation: Reduction Techniques and Immobilization
    - Proximal Tibiofibular Joint Dislocation

11. Soft Tissue Injuries of the Knee
    - Medial and Lateral Collateral Ligament Injuries
    - Grading and Management of Ligamentous Injuries

12. Management of Patellar Fractures
    - Clinical Assessment and Radiological Differentiation
    - Conservative and Surgical Treatment Approaches

13. Clinical Recommendations for Knee Injury Management
    - Imaging and Early Reassessment Protocols

- Reduction and Vascular Assessment for Dislocations
- Key Strategies for Preventing Long-Term Disability

Chapter 9 (I): Tibial Shaft Fractures and Ankle Joint Injuries

1. Tibial Shaft Fractures
   - Overview
   - Most common long bone fractures
   - High-energy trauma and associated soft tissue damage
   - Complications: Compartment syndrome, malunion, non-union
2. Mechanisms of Injury
   - High-energy trauma vs. torsional forces
   - Fracture patterns: Transverse, oblique, spiral, comminuted
3. Classification and Clinical Assessment
   - Classification
   - Skin integrity: Open vs. closed
   - Location: Proximal, middle, distal

- Type: Transverse, oblique, spiral, comminuted
- Angulation and displacement
- Clinical Assessment
- Pain, weight-bearing inability
- Neurovascular evaluation
- Associated injuries

4. Management and Compartment Syndrome
- Pain relief, reduction, immobilization
- Recognition and management of compartment syndrome
- Symptoms: Pain, diminished sensation, pulse loss
- Diagnostic

5. Radiological Evaluation and Definitive Management
- Imaging: AP and lateral radiographs
- Conservative vs. operative treatment
- Intramedullary nailing advantages

6. Specific Conditions
- Tibial Tubercle Fractures
- Classification (Watson-Jones)

- Conservative vs. surgical treatment
- Osgood-Schlatter Disease
- Differentiation and conservative management
- Tibial Stress Fractures
- Diagnosis and rest-based management

7. Ankle Joint Injuries
   1. Anatomy Overview
      - Bony and ligamentous structure
      - Role in stability and mobility
   2. Clinical Assessment
      - History
      - Injury mechanism, weight-bearing ability
      - Swelling and deformity evaluation
      - Examination
      - Palpation of bones, ligaments, and tendons
      - Range of motion and ligament stability tests
   3. Radiological Evaluation
      - Imaging: Standard X-rays, CT, MRI
      - Ottawa Ankle Rules: Indications for imaging

4. Ankle Fracture Classification Systems
- Weber Classification: Types A, B, C
- Henderson/Pott Classification: Unimalleolar, bimalleolar, trimalleolar
5. Management of Fractures
- Non-displaced fractures: Conservative management
- Displaced fractures: Open reduction and internal fixation (ORIF)
6. Special Fracture Types
- Tibial plafond (pilon) fractures
- Maisonneuve fractures
7. Ankle Dislocations
- Closed vs. open dislocations
- Reduction and surgical management
8. Soft Tissue Injuries
- Ligamentous injuries: Sprains and grades
- Achilles tendon rupture: Diagnosis and management

Chapter 9 (J) : Foot Injuries
1. Anatomy

- Overview of Foot Structure
- Hindfoot, Midfoot, Forefoot
- Subtalar, Midtarsal, and Tarsometatarsal Joints

2. Clinical Assessment
   - History
   - Trauma Types: Direct vs. Indirect
   - Key Symptoms: Pain, Swelling, Deformity
   - Examination
   - Limb Comparison, Palpation of Key Structures
   - Active and Passive Movements
   - Circulation and Neurological Assessment

3. Radiology
   - Routine Imaging Views
   - Ottawa Ankle and Foot Rules
   - Indications for X-rays
   - Additional Imaging
   - MRI for Stress Fractures
   - CT for Detailed Foot Imaging

4. Hindfoot Injuries
   - Calcaneal Fractures

- Mechanism, Classification, and Diagnosis
- Bohler Angle and CT Imaging
- Management: Conservative vs. Surgical
- Talar Fractures
- Mechanism and Classification
- Talar Neck and Dome Fractures
- Management of Talar Fractures

5. Lisfranc Injuries
- Diagnosis and Referral to Orthopedic Specialist
- Management: Closed Reduction and Fixation

6. Forefoot Fractures and Dislocations
- Metatarsal Shaft Fractures
- Mechanism, Diagnosis, and Management
- Hallux (Great Toe) Fractures
- Management: Nondisplaced vs. Displaced
- Base of Fifth Metatarsal Fractures

- Types: Tuberosity vs. Jones Fractures
- Management and Surgical Considerations

7. Metatarsophalangeal (MTP) Joint Dislocations
- Common Injuries: Fifth MTP, First MTP Dislocations
- Management: Reduction Techniques and Post-Reduction Care

8. Phalangeal Fractures and Dislocations
- Common Causes: Direct Trauma
- Management: Buddy Strapping, Displaced Fractures, and IP Joint Care

Chapter 9 (K) - Osteomyelitis: A Comprehensive Overview

1. Introduction
- Overview of osteomyelitis and its significance in emergency care.

2. Aetiology, Pathogenesis, and Pathology
- Haematogenous spread in children vs. adults

- Common pathogens and affected sites
- Pathophysiological changes in bone
- Development of abscesses, sequestra, and involucrum

3. Epidemiology
- Prevalence of osteomyelitis in healthy adults
- Influence of MRSA and regional variations (e.g., tuberculosis)

4. Clinical Features
- Common symptoms: localized pain, fever, swelling
- Differences in presentation by age group
- Specific signs in diabetic and pediatric patients

5. Risk Factors
- Surgery, trauma, diabetes, vascular disease
- Immunosuppression, intravenous drug use, and sickle cell disease

6. Examination
- Physical signs of infection: tenderness, warmth, swelling

- Specific presentations in elderly and diabetic patients

7. Investigations
   - Laboratory tests: WBC count, ESR, CRP, blood cultures
   - Imaging: X-rays, MRI, CT scans

8. Differential Diagnosis
   - Conditions to rule out

9. Management
   - Multidisciplinary approach: surgery, antibiotic therapy
   - Antibiotics for staphylococcal infections, MRSA considerations
   - Role of surgical intervention in chronic osteomyelitis

10. Prognosis
    - Impact of underlying conditions and infection site
    - Challenges in treating chronic osteomyelitis and potential for squamous cell carcinoma

11. Prevention
    - Infection control, surgical prevention, and

managing diabetic foot infections

12. Summary
- Key takeaways on osteomyelitis diagnosis, treatment, and outcomes

List of Abbreviations

ABG – Arterial Blood Gas

ACLS – Advanced Cardiovascular Life Support

AED – Automated External Defibrillator

BP – Blood Pressure

CBC – Complete Blood Count

CPR – Cardiopulmonary Resuscitation

CT – Computed Tomography

DVT – Deep Vein Thrombosis

ECG/EKG – Electrocardiogram

EMS – Emergency Medical Services

ESR – Erythrocyte Sedimentation Rate

GCS – Glasgow Coma Scale

ICU – Intensive Care Unit

IV – Intravenous

MRI – Magnetic Resonance Imaging

NPO – Nil Per Os (nothing by mouth)

PE – Pulmonary Embolism

PO – Per Os (by mouth)

PT – Prothrombin Time

PTT – Partial Thromboplastin Time

ACS – Acute Coronary Syndrome

ARDS – Acute Respiratory Distress Syndrome

ATLS – Advanced Trauma Life Support

CRP – C-Reactive Protein

FAST – Focused Assessment with Sonography for Trauma

MRSA – Methicillin-Resistant Staphylococcus aureus

NSTEMI – Non-ST Elevation Myocardial Infarction

PALS – Pediatric Advanced Life Support

ROSC – Return of Spontaneous Circulation

STEMI – ST-Elevation Myocardial Infarction

TBI – Traumatic Brain Injury

ASA – Acetylsalicylic Acid (Aspirin)

ETT – Endotracheal Tube

IVF – Intravenous Fluids

NGT – Nasogastric Tube

NSAID – Non-Steroidal Anti-Inflammatory Drug

TPA – Tissue Plasminogen Activator

CXR – Chest X-Ray

LFT – Liver Function Test

RFT – Renal Function Test
SpO$_2$ – Peripheral Oxygen
Saturation
CDC – Centers for Disease
Control and Prevention
PPE – Personal Protective
Equipment

Introduction

A well-developed emergency
medical system is crucial for
ensuring an effective response
during natural disasters and
humanitarian crises. Recently,
the World Health Organization
has emphasized the importance
of building emergency care
infrastructure and providing
essential training in low- and
middle-income countries.
Emergency medicine, once
viewed as a costly supplement
to essential healthcare, is now
recognized as a vital
component for disaster
preparedness and response.

Scope of Practice
The broad skill set of
emergency physicians enables
them to address a wide range of
medical issues, adapting to the
needs of diverse populations.
Although core competencies in
diagnosis and resuscitation are

universal, practice varies according to regional demands. In some under-resourced regions, emergency physicians may require proficiency in obstetrics, including cesarean sections, while others in urban centers may focus more on managing substance abuse cases or elderly care. The fundamental role of an emergency physician remains constant: to identify and address life- or limb-threatening conditions, establish priorities, diagnose and treat, and decide on either discharge or inpatient admission. Additionally, emergency physicians coordinate both clinical teams and systems to ensure high-quality patient care.

Emergency medicine has expanded to encompass numerous subspecialties, including toxicology, pediatrics, trauma, critical care, prehospital/disaster medicine, sports medicine, hyperbaric medicine, and academic emergency medicine. Specialized fellowships, typically lasting one to two years, are available in most of these fields. Nonetheless, all emergency physicians must acquire foundational knowledge across these areas to confidently handle unanticipated cases. In larger facilities with extensive specialist staff, these subspecialty skills enhance clinical service development and patient outcomes.

The Future

Emergency medicine has evolved from a small-scale practice to an integral, process-oriented system of healthcare, and this evolution will likely accelerate. Advances in diagnostics, treatment options, patient demographics, and collaborative healthcare approaches will shape the future of emergency medicine. Patients now expect more involvement in care decisions, faster access to services, and greater accountability from providers.

Potential challenges to emergency care quality include overemphasis on time-based performance metrics used to meet governmental targets, which can detract from patient care. Overcrowded emergency departments and recent changes in healthcare funding that limit access for low-income patients present further difficulties. Nonetheless, these challenges may also offer opportunities to refine care delivery and strengthen interdisciplinary collaboration. Emergency physicians play a crucial role in advocating for improvements in acute care systems. Despite obstacles, the specialty's core strength—providing consistent, high-quality care to diverse emergency patients at all times—underscores its value. By focusing on this mission, emergency medicine will continue to thrive and remain a central element of healthcare systems worldwide.

Chapter 1
Introduction to Basic Life Support (BLS)

Basic Life Support (BLS) is a critical emergency intervention focused on maintaining breathing and circulation in individuals experiencing cardiac arrest. The primary component of BLS is cardiopulmonary resuscitation (CPR), which emphasizes chest compressions and may include rescue breaths, generally without advanced equipment. BLS can be administered immediately by virtually any individual, even those with minimal training, guided by emergency dispatcher instructions, particularly in out-of-hospital cardiac arrest (OHCA) scenarios. Evidence consistently demonstrates the role of BLS in improving survival rates and preserving neurological function in patients with cardiac arrest.

This chapter provides a framework for BLS that any rescuer can perform while awaiting the arrival of emergency medical services (EMS) or advanced life support (ALS) personnel.

Essentials of Basic Life Support

1. Activation of the Chain of Survival: In cases of OHCA, rapid activation of the Chain of

Survival, including high-quality CPR and early defibrillation, is essential. Emergency dispatchers play a crucial role in guiding lay rescuers.

2. Dispatcher Assistance: Dispatchers should instruct callers on how to provide chest compressions-only CPR. This approach improves bystander CPR rates and enhances survival outcomes.

3. Chest Compressions: Bystanders should perform compressions on any unresponsive individual with abnormal or absent breathing. Trained rescuers may also incorporate rescue breaths if capable and without compromising the quality of compressions.

4. Defibrillation in BLS: Training in early defibrillation is fundamental in BLS, as it is vital for terminating VF.

5. Public Access Defibrillation Programs: Implementing defibrillator access programs empowers minimally trained or untrained bystanders to use automated external defibrillators (AEDs) in public

spaces, further enhancing survival opportunities

Chain of Survival

The Chain of Survival refers to a sequence of essential actions for addressing sudden cardiac arrest. These steps start with recognizing the cardiac event and promptly activating EMS. Rapid initiation of high-quality CPR, focusing on effective chest compressions, followed by defibrillation, is essential, as it markedly enhances survival chances, particularly in cases of ventricular fibrillation (VF) during OHCA. Evidence supports that administering CPR and defibrillation within 3 to 5 minutes of collapse from VF can result in survival rates ranging from 49% to 75%. Notably, each minute of delay in defibrillation decreases survival likelihood by approximately 10-12%. The final stages in the Chain of Survival encompass ALS and coordinated post-resuscitation care to sustain cardiac and neurological functions.

Development of Protocols

Evidence-based BLS protocols are developed to ensure consistency and effectiveness across diverse providers. Many countries have established national committees to create and endorse BLS guidelines for EMS, medical professionals, and the general public. The International Liaison Committee on Resuscitation (ILCOR), which includes organizations such as the American Heart Association (AHA) and the European Resuscitation Council (ERC), regularly reviews scientific advancements in BLS and ALS to update guidelines, with meetings every five years to consider recent research.

Organizations such as the American Heart Association (AHA), the European Resuscitation Council (ERC), and other international committees are part of ILCOR and provide guidelines tailored to regional needs.

DRSABCD Approach

The DRSABCD protocol (Dangers, Responsive, Send for help, Airway, Breathing, CPR,

Defibrillator) is a systematic BLS process for assessing and supporting a collapsed patient. This method involves:

- Assessing for potential dangers and responsiveness.
- Sending help immediately.
- Ensuring a clear airway and checking for abnormal breathing.
- Initiating CPR and applying a defibrillator as soon as possible.

Adult BLS Sequence

A major shift in adult BLS recommended by ILCOR was the adoption of a Compressions, Airway, Breathing (CAB) sequence to prioritize rapid initiation of chest compressions. This contrasts with the traditional Airway, Breathing, Compressions (ABC) sequence and aims to reduce delays, particularly in cases of witnessed, likely cardiac-origin arrests.

Regional Adaptations

Variations exist in BLS protocols between regions. For

instance, the ERC and the Australian Resuscitation Council (ARC) continue to emphasize opening the airway before checking breathing, maintaining an ABC approach to reduce confusion. Conversely, the AHA adheres to the CAB sequence.

Response Assessment

Upon discovering a collapsed individual, rescuers are encouraged to assess for unresponsiveness through basic methods like calling out and gently shaking the person. If unresponsive, the rescuer should immediately contact EMS, begin chest compressions, and follow dispatcher instructions.

In cases of suspected airway blockage, hypoxia, or conditions like drowning, trained responders may initiate CPR with ventilation before activating EMS.

Airway and Breathing Assessment

Rescuers assess the airway by checking for obstructions and using maneuvers like the head tilt–chin lift to open the airway, especially for trained personnel. In suspected trauma cases, spinal precautions are taken. Adequate breathing is assessed visually through chest movements and sounds. If breathing is abnormal or absent, the individual should be positioned safely in a lateral recovery position, maintaining open airways until EMS arrives.

Cardiopulmonary Resuscitation (CPR)

The current BLS recommendations prioritize immediate chest compressions over ventilations to minimize delays. Lay and healthcare rescuers are advised to perform compressions on the lower half of the sternum at a depth of at least 5 cm, at 100-120 compressions per minute. Full chest recoil between compressions and minimal interruptions are critical for effective CPR.

Incorporating Ventilation in CPR

For rescuers skilled in CPR with ventilation, a 30:2 compression-to-ventilation ratio is recommended, with breaths administered in under 10 seconds to avoid interrupting compressions.

Airway Management and Cardiac Arrest Response

During cardiac arrest in healthcare settings, basic airway devices can assist in effective early airway resuscitation (EAR). These tools, such as a simple face mask or bag-valve-mask (BVM) ventilation, may be used with or without an oropharyngeal Guedel airway. Benefits of these devices include familiarity among medical staff, reduced infection risks, enhanced aesthetics, and supplemental oxygen delivery, though training is required for effective use. Regardless of the ventilation method, chest rise within one second serves as an indicator of adequate tidal volume. Current guidelines for adult cardiac arrest emphasize using the highest feasible oxygen concentration during CPR to alleviate tissue hypoxia, though any oxygen level is deemed acceptable under these circumstances.

Defibrillation Protocol

When a defibrillator becomes available, electrode pads should promptly be placed on the patient, and the device activated. Self-adhesive defibrillation pads offer safety, convenience, and effectiveness, leading to their preference over handheld paddles. It is essential to prioritize the safety of all rescuers and team members during defibrillator use and shock administration.

Shock Administration

Using an automated external defibrillator (AED) involves following voice prompts like "stand clear" and "press the button" if shockable rhythms are detected. When using a manual defibrillator, healthcare providers must select the appropriate energy level and deliver a shock when detecting a shockable rhythm, such as ventricular fibrillation (VF) or pulseless ventricular tachycardia (VT).

Minimizing Interruptions in Chest Compressions

To maximize the likelihood of resuscitation, chest compressions should resume immediately after each shock, regardless of the resultant rhythm. Interruptions for rhythm checks, shock delivery, and other pre/post-shock pauses should be limited to 10 seconds or less.

Modern biphasic defibrillators, as opposed to older monophasic versions, are more effective at treating ventricular arrhythmias at lower energy settings. However, studies have not conclusively shown improvements in neurological outcomes or survival to hospital discharge.

If the AED indicates that a shock is unnecessary, rescuers should continue CPR with a 30:2 compression-to-ventilation ratio until professional assistance arrives or the patient exhibits signs of responsiveness.

Automated External Defibrillator Use

The AED is a core component of Basic Life Support (BLS). Designed for simplicity and safety, AEDs accurately identify VF and VT and can be used effectively by both trained and untrained rescuers in various settings.

Public-Access AED Programs

Research supports the placement of AEDs in public spaces, such as airports and sports facilities, enabling bystanders, minimally trained rescuers, and emergency responders to perform defibrillation during out-of-hospital cardiac arrest (OHCA). These programs have significantly improved survival rates, as evidenced by several national observational studies showing successful defibrillation and survival with public-access AEDs.

Home-Access AEDs

Home-access AEDs may be appropriate for patients at high risk of cardiac arrest who lack an implantable cardioverter-defibrillator (ICD). However, survival benefits from home AEDs have not been demonstrated conclusively, making their usage more of an individual choice rather than a general recommendation.

Implantable Cardioverter Defibrillators and CPR

ICDs, which deliver a 40 J shock to address arrhythmias, are used for patients with high cardiac arrest risk. While most patients remain conscious during defibrillation, CPR should begin if the patient loses consciousness and the ICD shocks fail to restore a stable rhythm. The ICD poses minimal risk to bystanders, though medical staff should wear gloves and minimize contact with the patient during device firing.

Summary of Basic Life Support Protocols

The "Chain of Survival" includes five critical steps for cardiac arrest management:

1. Immediate recognition and EMS activation,

2. Early CPR with emphasis on compressions,

3. Prompt defibrillation,

4. Advanced life support,

5. Integrated post-resuscitation care.

An unresponsive adult with irregular breathing should be assumed to have cardiac arrest, with trained rescuers applying the head tilt–chin lift method if necessary. Untrained rescuers should prioritize initiating compressions and activating EMS immediately. Resuscitation should continue until advanced support arrives, the patient recovers, or conditions prevent continued CPR.

Controversies and Unresolved Issues

Controversial topics include:

Choice between ABC or CAB sequence for initial CPR steps,

Role of passive oxygenation during compression-only CPR,

Bundled EMS interventions for non-shockable OHCA rhythms,

Ideal CPR cycle timing and rhythm check intervals,

Pulse checks during CPR in BLS,

Value of real-time audiovisual feedback and prompt devices during CPR.

Rhythm Recognition

1. Ventricular Fibrillation (VF)

VF is a chaotic, life-threatening rhythm without a detectable pulse. It features a disordered, irregular pattern with an undulating waveform, typically over 150 beats per minute. The ECG will show an inconsistent amplitude and morphology.

2. Pulseless Ventricular Tachycardia (VT)

Pulseless VT presents as wide, abnormally shaped ventricular complexes on the ECG, with no effective cardiac output. The heart rate generally exceeds 100 beats per minute and often surpasses 150, meeting the criteria for pulseless VT.

3. Asystole

Asystole is characterized by a complete absence of electrical activity on the ECG. Misinterpretation as "apparent asystole" can occur if:

ECG leads are disconnected or broken (indicated by electrical artifacts during chest compressions).

The ECG sensitivity is too low; increasing sensitivity might reveal artifacts.

Coarse VF may mimic asystole if the VF axis is perpendicular to the selected ECG lead. Checking at least two leads, preferably in perpendicular positions, is advised to confirm asystole.

4. Pulseless Electrical Activity (PEA)

PEA is when organized electrical activity is present without a detectable pulse. An arterial line, end-tidal CO_2 monitoring, or cardiac ultrasound can differentiate true PEA from pseudo-PEA. PEA generally has a poor prognosis, with lower survival rates compared to shockable rhythms. Observational studies have found better outcomes with electrical frequencies above 60 beats per minute in PEA patients.

Defibrillation Overview

Defibrillation is the only effective intervention for VF and pulseless VT. The defibrillator should be immediately available and a shock delivered without delay.

Pad/Paddle Positions: Two standard positions maximize defibrillation efficacy:

Anteroapical Position: One pad/paddle to the right of the sternum below the clavicle, the other at the cardiac apex along the mid-axillary line.

Anteroposterior Position: One pad/paddle on the precordium, with the other on the back near the spine at the scapula level.

Avoid placing defibrillation pads over ECG electrodes, medicated patches, or significant breast tissue. If the patient has an implanted device (e.g., pacemaker), keep pads at least 8 cm away and check device function after defibrillation.

Waveforms and Energy Levels

Modern defibrillators use biphasic waveforms with impedance compensation, which allows effective defibrillation at lower energy and minimizes post-shock ECG changes. Recommended initial energy for biphasic defibrillators is 150-200 J, with subsequent shocks at increased energy levels if possible. Older monophasic defibrillators, which use a sinusoidal waveform, require higher energy levels (typically 360 J for adults).

Optimizing Transthoracic Impedance

Successful defibrillation requires synchronous depolarization of a significant myocardial mass. Impedance can be reduced by:

Using conductive pads or electrode paste/gel, which reduces impedance by up to 30%.

Applying firm paddle pressure (5-8 kg) when adhesive pads are not used.

Defibrillating during expiration, when chest impedance is lower.

Automated External Defibrillators (AEDs)

AEDs, first introduced in 1979, are now standard equipment for emergency medical services (EMS) and public spaces. AEDs simplify defibrillation, allowing for rapid intervention by both trained professionals and lay responders in community settings. This rapid access to defibrillation can be critical, with community AED programs proving effective in improving survival rates.

Shock Delivery Protocol

When a shockable rhythm (VF or pulseless VT) is identified, the defibrillator should be charged during ongoing CPR. After ensuring no contact with the patient, a shock is administered, followed by an immediate resumption of CPR for two minutes without delay for rhythm analysis.

Technical Issues and Complications

If defibrillation fails to produce visible skeletal muscle contraction, ensure proper contact, defibrillator functionality, and adequate device settings. Common complications include:

Skin burns, minimized by ensuring good contact.

Potential myocardial injury or post-shock dysrhythmias with high-energy shocks.

Skeletal injuries, though rare, and risks to rescuers if accidental contact occurs during defibrillation.

Code Blue Process for Shockable Rhythms

Immediate defibrillation is critical for shockable rhythms (VF/pulseless VT), supported by brief intervals of CPR to improve myocardial and cerebral viability. Immediate post-shock CPR is essential, as cardiac function may be impaired, and a pulse may not be immediately palpable even after successful defibrillation.

Cardiac Arrest Medication Guidelines

Indications for Amiodarone

Persistent ventricular fibrillation (VF) or pulseless ventricular tachycardia (VT) despite defibrillation and adrenaline.

Prevention of recurrent VF or VT.

Side Effects of Amiodarone

May lead to low blood pressure, slow heart rate, heart block, and QTc prolongation, which can increase the risk of arrhythmias.

Dosage of Amiodarone

Initial bolus of 300 mg (or 5 mg/kg), with an additional 150 mg if needed.

Atropine

Atropine is no longer routinely recommended for asystole or pulseless electrical activity (PEA) due to inconsistent benefits in cardiac arrest.

Calcium Use

Indicated in cardiac arrest when caused or worsened by:

High potassium levels (hyperkalemia)

Low calcium levels (hypocalcemia)

Calcium channel blocker toxicity

Adverse Effects of Calcium

May increase cell death, leading to potential injury to the heart and brain.

Risk of tissue damage if there is leakage from the vein.

Calcium Dosage

5–10 mL of 10% calcium chloride or 15–30 mL of 10% calcium gluconate.

Lignocaine (Lidocaine)

Effective as an antiarrhythmic for survival to hospital discharge in VF cases, especially when amiodarone is unavailable.

Indications for Lignocaine

For VF or pulseless VT unresponsive to defibrillation

and adrenaline, or for recurrent VF/VT when amiodarone cannot be administered.

Side Effects of Lignocaine

May cause low blood pressure, bradycardia, heart block, asystole, as well as central nervous system disturbances (e.g., tremors, seizures, coma).

Lignocaine Dosage

Initial dose of 1–1.5 mg/kg with a repeat dose of 0.5 mg/kg after 5–10 minutes if necessary.

Magnesium Use

Used in cardiac arrest related to:

Torsades de pointes

Low potassium or magnesium levels

Digoxin toxicity

VF/VT not responding to defibrillation and adrenaline

Adverse Effects of Magnesium

High doses may cause muscle weakness or paralysis.

Magnesium Dosage

5 mmol bolus, with a follow-up infusion of 20 mmol over 4 hours.

Potassium

Administered only for hypokalemia-related cardiac arrest.

Side Effects of Potassium

Can cause hyperkalemia, leading to rhythm disturbances, and tissue necrosis if extravasation.

Potassium Dosage

5 mmol IV bolus.

Sodium Bicarbonate

Indicated only in cases of cardiac arrest caused or complicated by:

Hyperkalemia

Tricyclic antidepressant overdose

Severe metabolic acidosis

Cardiac arrest lasting beyond 15 minutes

Side Effects of Sodium Bicarbonate

May lead to metabolic alkalosis, hypernatremia, and hyperosmolality; CO_2 production may worsen acidosis.

Sodium Bicarbonate Dosage

1 mmol/kg (1 mL/kg of an 8.4% solution) over 2–3 minutes, adjusted by blood gas measurements.

Vasopressin

An alternative to adrenaline, though evidence for routine use is insufficient.

Adverse Effects of Vasopressin

Can cause cerebral edema, ongoing vasoconstriction, which may worsen myocardial ischemia and impair ventricular function, and a procoagulant effect.

Vasopressin Dosage

Single 40 U IV bolus during cardiac arrest.

Monitoring During CPR

1. End-Tidal CO2 (ETCO2)

Monitoring ETCO2 can assess CPR effectiveness, with values under 10 mmHg indicating poor perfusion. A rise in ETCO2 after return of spontaneous circulation (ROSC) is a positive indicator.

2. Arterial Blood Gases (ABGs)

Used to evaluate oxygenation and ventilation but may not accurately reflect tissue acidosis. Should not interrupt CPR.

Post-Resuscitation Care

A structured post-resuscitation protocol enhances survival. Key components include:

Targeted temperature management (32–36°C)

Advanced airway support

Normocapnia and target oxygen saturation (94–98%)
Seizure control and blood glucose management
Extracorporeal CPR (ECPR)
May improve survival when standard CPR fails, especially in facilities equipped for it.
Prognosis and Decision Points
ROSC within 25 minutes without intervention is unlikely in unwitnessed, unresponsive out-of-hospital cardiac arrest with no shocks or CPR. Prolonged ALS (>30 minutes) without ROSC generally indicates low survival likelihood, except in special cases (e.g., hypothermia).
Best Survival Chances
Best prognosis involves witnessed collapse, immediate CPR, shockable rhythm (VF or pulseless VT), and defibrillation within 2–3 minutes.

References

1. Nolan, J. P., Hazinski, M. F., Aickin, R., et al. (2015). Part 1: Executive Summary - 2015 International Consensus on Cardiopulmonary Resuscitation and Emergency Cardiovascular

Care Science and Treatment Recommendations.
Resuscitation, 95, e1–e31.
2. Cummins, R. O., Ornato, J. P., Thies, W. H., & Pepe, P. E. (1991). Enhancing Survival from Sudden Cardiac Arrest: The Chain of Survival Concept. A Statement for Health Professionals by the Advanced Cardiac Life Support Subcommittee and the Emergency Cardiac Care Committee, American Heart Association. Circulation, 83(5), 1832–1847.
3. Travers, A. H., Perkins, G. D., Berg, R. A., et al. (2015). Part 3: Adult Basic Life Support and Automated External Defibrillation - 2015 International Consensus on Cardiopulmonary Resuscitation and Emergency Cardiovascular Care Science and Treatment Recommendations. Circulation, 132(16 Suppl 1), S51–S83.
4. Beck, B., Bray, J., Cameron, P., et al. (2018). Regional Differences in Characteristics, Incidence, and Outcomes of Out-of-Hospital Cardiac Arrest in Australia and New Zealand:

Findings from the Aus-ROC Epistry. Resuscitation, 126, 49–57.

5. Wang, P. L., & Brooks, S. C. (2018). Mechanical Versus Manual Chest Compressions for Cardiac Arrest. Cochrane Database of Systematic Reviews, (8), Cd007260.

6. Flato, U. A., Paiva, E. F., Carballo, M. T., et al. (2015). Echocardiographic Assessment for Prognostication in ICU Patients with Non-Shockable Rhythm Cardiac Arrest During Resuscitation. Resuscitation, 92, 1–6.

7. Hagihara, A., Hasegawa, M., Abe, T., et al. (2012). Prehospital Epinephrine Use and Survival Outcomes in Out-of-Hospital Cardiac Arrest Cases. JAMA, 307(11), 1161–1168.

8. Perkins, G. D., Ji, C., Deakin, C. D., Quinn, T., Nolan, J. P., Scomparin, C., et al. (2018). A Randomized Controlled Trial of Epinephrine Administration in Out-of-Hospital Cardiac Arrest. New England Journal of Medicine, 379(8), 711–721.

9. Chowdhury, A., Fernandes, B., Melhuish, T. M., & White, L. D. (2018). A Systematic Review and Meta-Analysis of Antiarrhythmic Agents in Cardiac Arrest. Heart, Lung and Circulation, 27(3), 280–290.

10. Khan, S. U., Winnicka, L., Saleem, M. A., Rahman, H., & Rehman, N. (2017). Comparative Analysis of Amiodarone, Lidocaine, Magnesium, and Placebo in Shock-Refractory Ventricular Arrhythmia Using a Bayesian Network Meta-Analysis. Heart & Lung: The Journal of Acute and Critical Care, 46(6), 417–424.

11. Sasson, C., Hegg, A. J., Macy, M., et al. (2008). Prehospital Termination of Resuscitation in Refractory Out-of-Hospital Cardiac Arrest Cases. JAMA, 300(12), 1432–1438.

Chapter 2
Critical Care Management: Focused Overview with Detailed Airway and Ventilation Protocols

1. Airway Management and Ventilation

Effective airway assessment and ventilation management are pivotal in emergency and critical care. To address the risks associated with securing an airway, especially in rapid sequence intubation (RSI), the approach should prioritize patient stabilization and risk minimization.

Key Steps in Initial Airway Management:

Assessment: Initial assessment employs a "look, listen, feel" approach to quickly detect airway obstructions. Standard maneuvers, such as jaw thrust, chin lift, and head tilt, may be employed for basic clearance.

Clearance of Obstructions: In cases where foreign bodies obstruct the airway, a laryngoscope can assist in visualizing the obstruction, followed by the use of a Yankauer suction for fluids or Magill's forceps for solid items.

Oxygen Support: Upon airway clearance, oxygen administration via a face mask ensures adequate oxygenation as the team evaluates the patient's respiratory status.

2. Breathing Evaluation and Oxygenation

Breathing assessment continues with a "look, listen, feel" approach, aided by pulse oximetry to monitor oxygen saturation. Further assessment with arterial or venous blood gasses can provide insights into CO_2 levels.

Non-Invasive Ventilation (NIV): For patients with respiratory failure, especially those with hypoxemia or hypercapnia, NIV offers a controlled oxygen-air mixture through a positive pressure mask. This setup, typically maintaining pressure between 5–10 cm H_2O, improves oxygenation by enhancing alveolar recruitment.

BiPAP (Bi-level Positive Airway Pressure): For added inspiratory support, BiPAP may be indicated to reduce respiratory workload, particularly in patients with reduced lung compliance.

3. Essential Concepts in Critical Care

Common Presentations: Respiratory failure often requires immediate ventilatory support, with NIV as a primary intervention. For cases where NIV fails, endotracheal intubation and mechanical ventilation are necessary.

Rapid Sequence Intubation (RSI): This approach, involving sedatives and muscle relaxants, facilitates the placement of an endotracheal tube (ETT) safely and efficiently, reducing the risk of hypoxia.

Plan B for Difficult Airway Visualization: A contingency plan should be in place to manage cases where vocal cord visualization is challenging, ensuring patient safety against hypoxemia.

Verification of Tube Placement: Clinical assessments alone are unreliable for verifying tube placement. Waveform capnography remains the standard for confirming tracheal intubation.

Protective Ventilation Strategy: In patients with acute lung injury, low tidal volumes should be utilized to minimize barotrauma risk.

4. Contraindications and Considerations for NIV

NIV may be inappropriate for unresponsive or agitated patients, those intolerant to a tight face mask, or individuals with facial characteristics (like dense facial hair) that prevent an effective mask seal. Lack of trained personnel also poses a limitation.

5. Advanced Airway Management Protocol

Indications for RSI:

Airway Compromise: RSI is necessary for patients who cannot maintain airway patency or protection, especially unconscious patients at risk for aspiration.

Ventilatory Failure: Conditions requiring support range from traumatic injuries, such as flail chest, to systemic weaknesses, such as in Guillain-Barré syndrome.

Behavioral Management: Severely agitated patients

needing thorough examination and treatment may require sedation and airway management to enable safe clinical intervention.

Anticipated Deterioration: Patients with conditions prone to worsening, like head injuries or airway burns, benefit from proactive airway management to prevent escalation.

Pre-Procedure Preparation:

Assessment: A thorough pre-intubation assessment includes reviewing medications, allergies, and identifying any anatomical challenges.

Pre-oxygenation: A high concentration of oxygen is administered to reduce the risk of desaturation, allowing for a safer apneic period during intubation. Denitrogenation during this step helps maintain oxygen reserves in the lungs, lengthening the safe apnea window.

Apneic Oxygenation: For patients where rapid oxygen consumption may reduce safe apnea time (such as children or individuals with high metabolic demands), continuous high-flow nasal oxygen can extend the safe apnea period.

Controlled Face Mask Ventilation: In specific cases, such as profound hypoxia or acidosis, careful face mask ventilation is permissible to avoid hypoxia-related complications.

Intubation in Challenging Cases: For patients with agitation or those intolerant of pre-oxygenation, controlled administration of a muscle relaxant can facilitate the procedure.

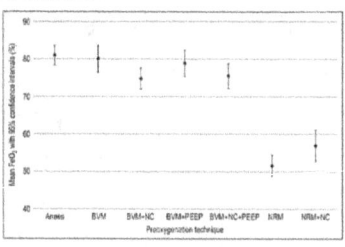

Figure 2-1 illustrates the average fraction of expired oxygen (FeO2) achieved with various preoxygenation methods, displaying results as mean values with a 95% confidence interval. Techniques compared include bag-valve-mask (BVM), nasal cannula (NC), non rebreather mask (NRM), and BVM with a positive end-expiratory pressure (PEEP) valve.

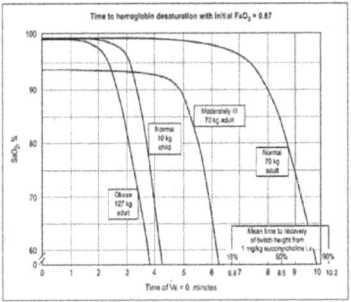

Figure 2-2 shows the relationship between oxygen saturation (SaO2) and apnoea duration across different patient types.

A rapid endotracheal intubation (ETI) approach is often linked to significant risks, including potential oxygen desaturation, even in normal airways. This risk intensifies in challenging airway cases. A safer strategy involves using sedation selectively to facilitate pre-oxygenation before performing Rapid Sequence Intubation (RSI), a method termed delayed sequence intubation (DSI). DSI acts as a procedural sedation technique that enhances pre-oxygenation. Ketamine, administered intramuscularly (IM) or intravenously (IV), is often recommended due to its ability to preserve airway patency and ventilation during sedation.

Patient Positioning

For trauma patients requiring spinal stabilization, positioning in reverse Trendelenburg can optimize ventilation-perfusion (V/Q) matching. A folded towel under the occiput aligns the cervical spine anatomically, improving the airway's position for both laryngoscopy and bag-valve-mask (BVM) ventilation. During intubation, manual in-line stabilization should be consistently applied. For patients without spinal concerns, positioning the head in an ear-to-sternal-notch alignment, with the face parallel to the ceiling, is often preferred.

Team and Equipment Preparation

A structured RSI checklist is crucial to ensure thorough preparation of the team, equipment, and patient. Using a standardized RSI setup or a "kit-dump" layout can also expedite equipment readiness. Essential preparations include pre-loading and labeling all medications, ensuring a backup laryngoscope, and opening, lubricating, and testing the primary and a size-smaller endotracheal tube (ETT). A bougie and a stylet to shape the ETT are also recommended for immediate accessibility. The airway team—typically a laryngoscopy and an airway assistant—should confirm readiness before administering RSI drugs.

Considerations for Cricoid Pressure

The application of cricoid pressure remains debated; while traditionally used to prevent aspiration, newer evidence suggests it may impair laryngoscopic visualization. Practitioners should evaluate its use based on current evidence.

Monitoring Protocols

Continuous monitoring during RSI should include electrocardiography (ECG), pulse oximetry, and blood pressure assessment. Hemodynamically unstable patients may require intra-arterial blood pressure monitoring. Additionally, calibrated waveform capnography is essential for accurate end-tidal CO_2 ($ETCO_2$) measurement post-intubation.

Airway Pharmacology

The optimal sedative agent for RSI would rapidly induce unconsciousness, amnesia, and analgesia while preserving cerebral perfusion and avoiding major hemodynamic disturbances. However, no single drug perfectly meets these criteria. Sedative choices include:

Ketamine: Known for its dissociative anesthesia properties, ketamine offers analgesia and maintains airway reflexes and respiratory drive. It may also increase heart rate, blood pressure, and cardiac output, making it beneficial for patients in shock, traumatic brain injuries, or severe asthma. However, caution is warranted in patients with coronary artery disease or uncontrolled hypertension.

Propofol: This short-acting anesthetic has rapid onset but

may cause significant hypotension, which limits its use in hemodynamically unstable patients.

Thiopentone: Effective for quick, deep sedation and useful in lowering intracranial pressure, thiopentone also has anticonvulsant properties but can depress myocardial function, so caution is required in patients with shock or on beta-blockers.

Midazolam: A benzodiazepine option, though its slower onset may reduce its efficacy for emergency RSI use.

Paralytic Agents

Suxamethonium (succinylcholine) is often the first choice for RSI due to its rapid onset and short duration of action. Nevertheless, it carries risks such as bradycardia, hyperkalemia (especially in patients with recent burns or crush injuries), and masseter muscle spasm. In cases where muscle rigidity occurs, a non-depolarizing muscle relaxant like rocuronium may be used as an alternative.

Stepwise Technique for Endotracheal Intubation (ETI)

Performing endotracheal intubation (ETI) in a systematic manner enhances the visibility of the larynx and facilitates the smooth passage of the endotracheal tube (ETT). The process begins with suctioning the pharynx to clear any secretions. The laryngoscopy then carefully positions the laryngoscope blade at the base of the tongue to expose the uvula. The blade is gradually advanced, visualizing the epiglottis, and further inserted until the tip reaches the vallecula, engaging the hyoepiglottic ligament. Lifting the laryngoscope handle elevates the soft tissues and exposes the glottis, providing a clearer view of the vocal cords. If necessary, external laryngeal manipulation can be applied by the laryngoscopy, who uses their right hand to move the thyroid cartilage, optimizing the view. Additionally, slight elevation of the patient's head may improve the view in most cases.

Techniques to Improve Laryngoscopic View:

External laryngeal manipulation (removing cricoid pressure if applied)

Elevating the head

Adjusting the operator's position

Changing the patient's positioning

Altering the laryngoscope type

Suctioning excess secretions

Inserting the laryngoscope blade deep along the midline, then withdrawing it slowly to identify the correct anatomy.

The laryngoscopic view should be documented along with any maneuvers needed to achieve the desired visualization. Cormack and Lehane classified laryngoscopic views into grades 1–4, where:

Grade 1: Entire glottis is visible.

Grade 2: Only the posterior vocal cords or arytenoids are visible.

Grade 3: Only the epiglottis is visible.

Grade 4: Only the soft palate is visible.

In the emergency department (ED), a bougie or a stylet shaped for direct intubation is highly recommended for rapid sequence intubation (RSI) as these patients are often at risk for difficult intubation. When using a bougie, any resistance felt at the aryepiglottic fold can be overcome by rotating the ETT counterclockwise or using a smaller tube. Rotating the tube clockwise helps advance it over the stylet, reducing the risk of it catching on tracheal rings. Throughout this process, it is crucial to maintain visualization of the glottis to assist with tube passage and ensure continuous oxygenation during apnoeic periods.

Confirmation of Endotracheal Tube Placement

Successful tracheal intubation is confirmed through capnography or a colorimetric CO_2 detector. The presence of a normal capnography waveform indicates proper tube placement. If no waveform is detected, the intubation attempt has failed. Other signs of correct placement include visible misting of the ETT, stable oxygen saturation levels, and equal air entry into both lungs, although these can be less reliable. A chest X-ray (CXR) should be used to confirm that the ETT is positioned approximately 5 cm above the carina.

Complications of Rapid Sequence Intubation (RSI)

Hypotension is a common complication after ETI, resulting from sedative medications causing vasodilation or negative inotropic effects, and the reduction in preload from positive-pressure ventilation. This can be addressed with fluid resuscitation, such as administering a bolus of saline or Hartmann's solution, and/or by using vasopressors or inotropes depending on the clinical situation. In cases of bronchospasm, hypotension may be caused by gas trapping, which can be relieved by temporarily disconnecting the patient from the ventilator circuit to allow for prolonged expiration. Additionally, a tension pneumothorax may develop after initiating positive-pressure ventilation, causing hypoperfusion. Conversely, hypertension often suggests inadequate sedation and analgesia.

Face Mask Ventilation (FMV)

Effective FMV is essential for both pre-oxygenation and deoxygenation, although it can be challenging. The key to success is maintaining a tight mask seal and ensuring patent airway, which can be facilitated by jaw thrust and the use of airway adjuncts such as nasopharyngeal or oropharyngeal airways. Suctioning the pharynx and releasing cricoid pressure may also improve airway patency. A two-person technique is preferred: one person secures the mask and applies a jaw thrust, while the second person squeezes the bag with small tidal volumes at a slow rate (6–8 breaths per minute) to minimize gastric insufflation and mask leak. Proper positioning of the patient, as described earlier, also aids in effective FMV. The reverse Trendelenburg position may further assist by alleviating abdominal pressure on the diaphragm.

Supraglottic Airways (SGA)

SGA devices are often used as rescue devices in the ED. Although not a definitive airway, they offer protection against aspiration and typically provide higher airway pressures with less gastric insufflation than FMV. SGAs are typically used when intubation is unsuccessful or impractical.

Video-Laryngoscopy

The use of video-laryngoscopy for ETI is becoming increasingly common, as it provides real-time visualization and assists with external laryngeal manipulation. Video-laryngoscopy follows the same principles as direct laryngoscopy, but with the added advantage of visual guidance. Prior to insertion, the airway should be cleared of secretions to avoid obscuring the camera view. Hyper-angulated blades often provide excellent visualization of the larynx, but they may pose challenges when guiding the ETT between the vocal cords. A partial view, focusing on the posterior vocal cords and arytenoids, may provide a more effective guide for ETT placement. A stylet designed to fit the blade should always be used to facilitate proper tube positioning.

Front-of-Neck Access (FONA)

In cases of failed intubation, front-of-neck access (FONA) may be required. Surgical cricothyroidotomy is preferred over needle cricothyroidotomy because it allows for ventilation and airway protection. Percutaneous techniques are slower and less effective than the scalpel-finger-bougie approach. FONA is performed with the patient in an optimal position, with the neck extended and the larynx stabilized using the non-dominant hand. A vertical incision is made in the midline over the cricothyroid membrane, which is then incised horizontally. The index finger is inserted into the cricothyroid space, maintaining the tract and allowing passage of a bougie into the trachea. An ETT is then inserted over the bougie. In obese patients, a longer incision and blunt dissection may be required. Bleeding can obscure the anatomy, requiring reliance on palpation of the laryngeal structures.

Difficult Airway Management

Airway difficulty may arise due to anatomical or physiological factors, or human error. Anticipating difficult airways and preparing for them is vital. In ED patients, airway procedures are often more challenging due to unfasted status, underlying physiological derangements, or urgent circumstances. A comprehensive plan should be made and communicated to the team before proceeding with intubation. Algorithms for difficult airway management guide operators through a systematic approach when standard techniques fail. It is essential to optimize positioning and physiology, ensure equipment availability, and formulate a tailored plan.

Difficult airway algorithms, such as those by the Difficult Airway Society or the Vortex Approach, provide a structured response during an airway crisis. Successful oxygenation remains the primary goal. Surgical airway should be considered promptly if less invasive techniques fail.

Factors Contributing to Anatomical Difficulty

Distorted anatomy from factors such as radiation, tumors, hematomas, or infections increases the likelihood of airway difficulties. In such cases, a fiberoptic or awake intubation approach may be appropriate, with a surgical airway backup available.

Burns and Airway Securing

Airway management in burn patients is critical, particularly in cases of hoarseness, stridor, or burns involving the face or mouth. Intubation should be performed by an experienced operator with a surgical airway backup ready. Delayed intubation or incorrect technique may lead to further complications.

Airway Trauma

Signs of airway trauma, including dyspnea, stridor, or subcutaneous emphysema, require careful airway management to avoid exacerbating the injury. In these cases, a surgical airway may be the safest option if traditional techniques are unsuccessful.

Credentialing in Airway Management

To provide optimal care during airway emergencies, airway practitioners across all disciplines must develop and maintain both technical and non-technical skills essential for safe and effective management. For emergency physicians, credentialing should focus on achieving proficiency in critical technical skills, such as laryngoscopy and cricothyroidotomy. This can be achieved through hands-on experience in the operating theater and specialized emergency airway courses. Furthermore, it is crucial that these practitioners develop an understanding of the human factors that contribute to difficult airway management, as well as strategies to ensure an effective team response in challenging situations.

References
1. Boldrini, R., Fasano, L., & Nava, S. (2012). Noninvasive mechanical ventilation. Current Opinion in Critical Care, 18(1), 48–53.

2. Groombridge, C., Chin, C. W., Hanrahan, B., & Holdgate, A. (2016). Evaluation of preoxygenation techniques in non-operating room environments. Academic Emergency Medicine, 23(3), 342–346.

3. Ramachandran, S. K., Cosnowski, A., Shanks, A., & Turner, C. R. (2010). Apneic oxygenation during prolonged laryngoscopy in obese patients: A randomized controlled trial on nasal oxygen use. Journal of Clinical Anesthesia, 22(3), 164–168.

4. Benumof, J. L., Dagg, R., & Benumof, R. (1997). Critical hemoglobin desaturation before recovery from paralysis after 1

mg/kg intravenous succinylcholine. Anesthesiology, 87(4), 979–982.

5. Weingart, S. D., Trueger, N. S., Wong, N., et al. (2015). Delayed sequence intubation: A prospective observational study. Annals of Emergency Medicine, 65(4), 349–355.

6. Lane, S., Saunders, D., Schofield, A., et al. (2005). Comparison of preoxygenation efficacy in 20-degree head-up versus supine position: A randomized controlled trial. Anaesthesia, 60(11), 1064–1067.

7. Levitan, R. M., Mechem, C. C., Ochroch, E. A., et al. (2003). Enhancing laryngeal exposure during laryngoscopy with head-elevated positioning. Annals of Emergency Medicine, 41(3), 322–330.

8. Lebowitz, P. W., Shay, H., Straker, T., et al. (2012). Improved laryngoscopic views with shoulder and head elevation in obese and non-obese patients. Journal of Clinical Anesthesia, 24(2), 104–108.

9. Bhatia, N., Bhagat, H., & Sen, I. (2014). Cricoid pressure: Current perspectives. Journal of Anaesthesiology Clinical Pharmacology, 30(1), 3–6.

10. Frerk, C., Mitchell, V. S., McNarry, A. F., et al. (2015). The Difficult Airway Society 2015 guidelines for managing unanticipated difficult intubations in adults. British Journal of Anaesthesia, 115(6), 827–848.

Chapter 3
Oxygen Therapy

Oxygen, a vital component of life, was first identified by Joseph Priestley in 1772 and later used therapeutically by Thomas Beddoes in 1794. Today, it remains a cornerstone of medical treatment. Oxygen makes up 21% of the atmosphere, and its presence is crucial for cellular function. A deficiency in oxygen can lead to cellular hypoxia, regardless of the underlying cause. Hypoxaemia, a condition characterized by reduced oxygen in the blood, can lead to anaerobic metabolism, which is inefficient and potentially fatal if not addressed. As such, the management of hypoxia is a primary focus in acute care, making oxygen the most frequently administered therapeutic agent in emergency medicine. The administration of supplemental oxygen has well-established physiological benefits for acutely ill and injured patients.

Uses of Supplemental Oxygen

Supplemental oxygen serves several purposes in clinical settings:

Improving airway clearance: A clear airway is essential to ensure that oxygen reaches the lungs effectively.

Enhancing pulmonary gas exchange: Oxygen is given to address insufficient blood oxygenation due to issues with pulmonary function.

Maximizing arterial oxygen saturation (SaO2): In cases where the cardiovascular system cannot transport enough oxygen, supplemental oxygen helps increase the SaO2.

Supporting oxygen delivery under increased demand:

Supplemental oxygen can increase the oxygen content in the blood when tissues require more oxygen due to stress or disease.

Providing 100% oxygen: In specific cases, such as carbon monoxide poisoning or cyanide toxicity, 100% oxygen is essential.

Titrating oxygen therapy: In patients with impaired respiratory response, oxygen dosage may be carefully adjusted based on clinical monitoring.

Physiology of Oxygen Transport

Oxygen transport to tissues occurs through several key stages:

1. Ventilation: The process of moving air into and out of the lungs to facilitate gas exchange.

2. Pulmonary gas exchange: Oxygen from the air diffuses across the alveolar membrane into the blood, while carbon dioxide moves in the opposite direction.

3. Oxygen transport in the blood: Oxygen binds to

hemoglobin (Hb), which carries it through the bloodstream.

4. Local tissue perfusion: The heart pumps oxygen-rich blood to tissues.

5. Diffusion at the tissue level: Oxygen moves from the blood into the cells, where it is used for cellular metabolism.

6. Tissue utilization of oxygen: Once inside the cells, oxygen is utilized for energy production.

Ventilation and Hypoxia

At sea level, the partial pressure of oxygen in inspired air (PIO2) is approximately 20 kPa (150 mm Hg). Hypoxia can result if there is a reduction in the fraction of inspired oxygen (FIO2), which occurs at high altitudes or in poorly ventilated areas. For example, on a commercial airplane at 2400 meters, the cabin pressure decreases, reducing the available oxygen to about 14.4 kPa (108 mm Hg). Several conditions can impair ventilation, including airway obstruction, respiratory muscle weakness, neurological disorders affecting respiratory drive (e.g., head injury), and chest trauma. These impairments reduce the partial pressure of oxygen in the alveoli, leading to insufficient oxygen in the blood.

The alveolar gas equation provides a means to estimate the oxygen partial pressure in the alveoli (PAO2):

Pulmonary Gas Exchange

Oxygen diffusion from the alveoli into the pulmonary capillaries occurs passively, driven by concentration gradients. The Fick law of diffusion explains the relationship between the rate of gas transfer (VO2), tissue area, and other factors. For healthy individuals, oxygen quickly transfers from the alveoli to the blood, typically saturating pulmonary capillary blood within 0.25 seconds. The expected difference between the alveolar and arterial oxygen partial pressures (A-a gradient) provides an indication of the efficiency of pulmonary gas exchange.

An increased A-a gradient suggests issues with diffusion, such as pulmonary fibrosis, edema, or ventilation/perfusion mismatch, which can impair oxygen uptake.

Oxygen Carriage in the Blood

Oxygen is carried in the blood primarily by hemoglobin, with a smaller portion dissolved in plasma. For instance, at sea level, oxygen dissolved in plasma amounts to 0.03 mL per liter of blood per mm Hg of PaO_2. When PaO_2 is 100 mm Hg, approximately 3 mL of oxygen is dissolved in plasma. The oxygen-carrying capacity of blood is significantly greater due to the binding of oxygen to hemoglobin. Under normal conditions, blood with a hemoglobin concentration of 150 g/L carries around 200 mL of oxygen per liter.

The Haemoglobin-Oxygen Dissociation Curve illustrates the relationship between the oxygen partial pressure (PaO_2) and the amount of oxygen bound to hemoglobin. A rightward shift in the curve (caused by factors like increased temperature, low pH, or high CO_2) facilitates the release of oxygen to tissues, while a leftward shift (due to conditions such as high pH or low CO2) favors oxygen binding.

Oxygen Flux and Delivery

The total oxygen delivered to the tissues per minute, or oxygen flux, is determined by both the oxygen bound to hemoglobin and the amount dissolved in plasma. The formula for oxygen flux takes into account hemoglobin concentration, arterial oxygen saturation (SaO2), and cardiac output:

In a healthy individual with a cardiac output of 5 L/min, approximately 1000 mL of oxygen is delivered per minute to tissues. However, this reserve can be compromised in illness or injury, requiring supplemental oxygen to maintain adequate tissue oxygenation.

Local Tissue Perfusion and Diffusion

Impaired tissue perfusion or diffusion increases the demand for oxygen. Conditions such as oedema, whether caused by medical conditions or injury, can increase the distance oxygen must diffuse to reach cells. This requires higher levels of oxygen in the blood to ensure adequate delivery.

Tissue Utilization of Oxygen

Increased tissue oxygen demands occur under various conditions, such as fever or infections (sepsis). Additionally, diseases that impair tissue oxygen utilization, such as mitochondrial disorders, may further increase the need for supplemental oxygen. Elevating cardiac output can help meet these increased demands, but this may be limited by the underlying disease process.

The oxygen delivery system's performance is determined by factors such as the minute volume of the patient, the flow rate, and the specific characteristics of the delivery system. These systems can be broadly classified into fixed-performance and variable-performance systems based on the level of oxygen concentration they provide.

Fixed-Performance Oxygen Delivery Systems

Fixed-performance systems deliver a specified fraction of inspired oxygen (FI_O2) that remains constant, irrespective of changes in the patient's respiratory rate, volume, or inspiratory flow rate. A subset of these systems, 100% oxygen delivery systems, guarantees the delivery of pure oxygen.

General Principles

In Australian and New Zealand emergency departments, oxygen is commonly supplied through wall-mounted flow meters that deliver up to 15 L/min. Most oxygen delivery systems are connected to these devices. A flow rate of 15 L/min is usually insufficient to meet the high oxygen demands of adults, especially in cases where the peak inspiratory flow rate (PIFR) exceeds the system's supply:

A quiet, resting adult typically has a PIFR between 30 to 40 L/min, which exceeds the supply from a 15 L/min system. Consequently, devices like the Hudson mask must mix in ambient air to match the patient's breathing rate, reducing the FI_O2 to a maximum of 0.6.

The minute respiratory volume (RMV) of an adult typically ranges from 4 to 8 L, and for children, it is roughly 150 mL/kg. Systems designed to store oxygen during expiration, such as those with a reservoir, enhance oxygen economy. However, if the minute volume surpasses the oxygen supply (e.g., greater than 15 L/min), there is a risk of hypoxia due to inadequate oxygen delivery or a drop in FI_O2 if safety valves are activated to admit air.

To address this, some systems provide flow rates up to 25 L/min. These can improve oxygen flow but may still be subject to variations in performance based on the patient's ventilation needs. Notably, children, due to their smaller ventilation requirements, can receive high FI_O2 from a standard 15 L/min oxygen source, unlike adults.

Oxygen delivery systems can be categorized by their efficiency in oxygen use and whether they can also serve to ventilate patients manually.

Variable-Performance Systems

These systems adjust the FI_O2 delivered based on factors such as the patient's respiratory pattern and inspiratory flow. Common variable-performance systems include:

1. Nasal Cannulae: Typically used at flow rates between 1-4 L/min, nasal cannulas deliver FI_O2 between 22% and 40%. They work by utilizing the patient's respiratory pause to increase oxygen delivery. However, their performance depends on the patient's breathing pattern. Nasal cannulas are particularly useful for stable COPD patients but are less effective in those with dyspnea due to excessive mouth breathing.

2. Face Masks (e.g., Hudson, Edinburgh, Medishield): These masks supply a small oxygen reservoir, but their effectiveness is limited by the patient's inspiratory flow rate.

At flow rates between 6-15 L/min, they deliver FI_O2 ranging from 35% to 60%. A reservoir bag attached to the mask can store oxygen during exhalation, enhancing efficiency, but it may also increase the risk of CO_2 rebreathing.

3. T Pieces and Y Connectors: These systems are typically used for humidified oxygen supply or to administer nebulized medications. However, they are inefficient, requiring high flow rates and leading to wastage of oxygen. Their use has largely been replaced by more advanced systems like oxygen blenders.

Fixed-Performance Systems

Two primary types of fixed-performance systems used in emergency departments are:

1. Venturi Masks: These masks deliver a fixed FI_O2 by entraining air through a venturi system. The oxygen concentration can be controlled by changing the adapter or dial on the mask, with FI_O2 values ranging from 0.24 to 0.60. They are most effective when the

total flow rate exceeds 60 L/min to prevent performance variability. Venturi masks are ideal for managing conditions like chronic obstructive pulmonary disease (COPD), providing stable oxygen levels and minimizing CO_2 rebreathing.

2. Oxygen Blenders: These devices combine oxygen with air from multiple sources to deliver a precise FI_O2 (from 0.21 to 1.0) and are capable of adding humidification. Oxygen blenders are especially useful in emergency settings where high flow rates are needed and are increasingly employed in the management of critically ill patients. However, their high cost and lack of portability can be a disadvantage.

One Hundred Percent Oxygen Delivery Systems

These systems are designed to deliver 100% oxygen and vary in their efficiency. The systems include:

Free-flowing Circuits: To deliver 100% oxygen, flow rates must exceed the patient's PIFR, often requiring multiple oxygen ports. However, this system is inefficient as it does not use oxygen economically.

Reservoir Systems: By storing oxygen during exhalation and using it during inspiration, these systems improve oxygen use efficiency. However, they require the reservoir volume to be greater than the patient's tidal volume to function effectively.

Demand Valve Systems: These systems deliver oxygen corresponding to the patient's minute volume without the need for a reservoir, offering more efficient oxygen use.

Closed-Circuit Systems: These are the most oxygen-efficient systems as they recycle exhaled CO_2, replacing it with low-flow fresh oxygen. This minimizes oxygen consumption significantly.

Here is the paraphrased and clarified version of the text, with simplified language and an improved structure while maintaining evidence-based analysis:

Manual Ventilation System:
Advantages:

Pressure Regulation: The operator controls the pressure during manual ventilation, which helps reduce gastric distension.

Portability: The system is compact and can be easily transported to the field.

Disadvantages:

Fresh Gas Flow Depletion: Once the fresh gas supply is exhausted, the circuit stops working.

Oxygen Dilution: Exhaled nitrogen from the patient's early breaths may enter the circuit, potentially lowering the fraction of inspired oxygen (FiO_2) below 1.0. This issue can be mitigated by periodically purging the reservoir.

CO_2 Accumulation: The soda lime canister can cause CO_2 buildup if it is old or malfunctioning.

Inhalation of Soda Lime Dust: While rare, improper handling of the soda lime canister could lead to the inhalation of dust.

Cumbersome Design: The reservoir bag is positioned far from the patient's mask, making the system harder to use.

Helium and Oxygen Mixtures (Heliox):

Over the past decade, the use of helium mixed with oxygen (Heliox) has garnered attention. The typical oxygen concentration in Heliox is 30%. Heliox has a lower density than air, which can help reduce airway resistance, especially in conditions like chronic obstructive pulmonary disease (COPD), asthma, and bronchiolitis. This lower density potentially reduces the work of breathing.

Mechanism: Helium (He) is lighter than nitrogen, so when combined with oxygen, it lowers the gas mixture's density, which can be beneficial when FiO_2 ranges from 0.2 to 0.4. However, this advantage diminishes with FiO_2 greater than 0.4.

Limitations: While Heliox has lower density, its viscosity is not significantly lower than that of air. The theoretical benefit is most notable in cases of turbulent gas flow, such as those seen in COPD and asthma, where there is both small and medium airway involvement.

Clinical Evidence: Despite its potential advantages, the clinical evidence for Heliox in treating COPD or asthma is not robust. Further studies are needed to establish its definitive role in these conditions.

Measurement of Oxygenation: Assessing oxygenation through clinical signs alone, such as cyanosis, is unreliable due to its variability based on factors like hemoglobin levels, skin pigmentation, and lighting. More accurate measurements are provided by arterial blood gasses (ABG) and pulse oximetry, which allow precise titration of oxygen therapy.

Pulse Oximetry: This is the most common and non-invasive tool for assessing oxygenation in emergency medicine. Pulse oximeters are referred to as the "fifth vital sign" because they offer real-time, continuous assessment of oxygen saturation (SaO2) and the patient's response to oxygen therapy. However, it is important to recognize that SaO2 alone is not an indicator of ventilatory function and cannot detect rising CO_2 levels until the patient's condition worsens. This is why patients with respiratory compromise or those under sedation should be carefully monitored with end-tidal CO_2 or ABG analysis. Recent studies suggest that a drop in SaO2 may precede CO_2 accumulation, particularly during procedural sedation in children.

Factors Affecting Pulse Oximetry: Understanding the hemoglobin-oxygen dissociation curve and factors that can interfere with oximeter readings is crucial for accurate interpretation.

Pediatric Oxygen Therapy:
The principles of oxygen therapy for children are similar to those for adults, but certain physiological and psychological factors must be considered.

Body Size Considerations: Children have smaller airways

and a higher metabolic rate, so increased dead space in equipment can lead to CO_2 retention. Moreover, children may struggle to tolerate increased ventilation resistance.

Oxygen Flow: Because of their smaller size, children require less oxygen flow to achieve high FiO_2 values. For example, a Hudson mask at 8 L/min may provide FiO_2 of 0.8 in young children.

Appropriate Equipment: The use of appropriately sized masks, probes, laryngoscopes, and endotracheal tubes is essential to avoid complications like barotrauma. Pediatric resuscitators are designed with pressure relief valves to protect against excessive pressure.

Jackson-Rees Circuit: This smaller Mapleson F circuit is suitable for both spontaneous and manual ventilation of children. By maintaining a fresh gas flow two to three times the minute volume, it prevents rebreathing of CO_2. The circuit's design allows the operator to observe bag movement and detect airway obstructions more effectively, though it requires skill and experience to use safely.

Psychological Factors: Children often experience anxiety during oxygen therapy, so having a parent present can help alleviate fear. A loose mask or directing oxygen at the child's face using a tube can be effective in these situations.

Oxygen Toxicity: Prolonged use of oxygen at FiO2 levels above 0.6 for more than 24 hours can lead to oxygen toxicity, particularly in infants. It is essential to monitor oxygen levels carefully to minimize this risk, though oxygen should not be withheld due to fear of toxicity.

Oxygen Therapy During Patient Transfer:

Supplemental oxygen is essential during patient transport, especially in air travel where reduced ambient pressure can exacerbate existing hypoxia. Patients with conditions like decompression illness or arterial gas embolism must be transported at cabin pressures of at least 101.3 kPa

(1 ATA) to prevent worsening of their condition.

Considerations for Transport: When planning oxygen therapy for patient transport, it is crucial to estimate the oxygen consumption, transport time, potential deterioration, and a safety margin of at least 50%. Closed circuits with CO_2 absorbers are the most economical for prolonged transport, while free-flowing circuits are less cost-effective.

Monitoring During Transport: Pulse oximetry is vital to detect hypoxia during transport. Alarms should be used to alert the medical team to any significant changes in oxygen saturation. Oxygen therapy should be adjusted according to SaO_2 levels, especially during air travel when oxygen partial pressure changes with altitude.

Oxygen Therapy in Specific Conditions:

1. Asthma:

In asthma, hypoxia is caused by ventilation/perfusion mismatches due to broncho-constriction, secretions, inflammation, and edema.

Oxygen should be titrated to maintain SaO2 above 90%, ideally around 94%, especially between doses of bronchodilators. If hypoxia persists, oxygen flow may need to be increased to 100%.

For mechanical ventilation in asthma, it is important to use FiO2 of 1.0, high inspiratory flow, and a low tidal volume to minimize risks like hyperinflation and barotrauma.

2. Chronic Obstructive Pulmonary Disease (COPD):

Many patients with COPD present in acute respiratory failure, which may result from infection, bronchospasm, or other complications. Oxygen therapy should aim for an SaO2 of 88-90%. Blood gas analysis is key to adjusting oxygen levels, particularly for patients with impaired ventilatory responses to CO2.

In clinical practice, oxygen therapy must be carefully managed to avoid complications while achieving an optimal balance between oxygenation and carbon dioxide levels. For patients with chronic obstructive pulmonary disease (COPD), oxygen saturation should be maintained within a target range of 88% to 92%. When saturation falls below 90%, the oxygen dissociation curve steepens, making small increases in oxygen effective unless a pulmonary shunt is present. Therefore, initial oxygen therapy (FIO_2 of 0.24–0.28) is administered and adjusted based on the patient's response.

A repeat blood gas sample should be taken after 10 minutes of oxygen administration. This helps to monitor the partial pressure of carbon dioxide ($PaCO_2$), as the Haldane effect may cause a slight rise in $PaCO_2$. If this increase exceeds 1–1.3 kPa (8–10 mm Hg), it indicates an impaired ventilatory response to CO_2. In this case, the oxygen dose should be reduced incrementally until a satisfactory pulse oximetry reading is achieved while maintaining acceptable CO_2 levels. If the patient responds normally to CO2, there should be no significant rise in PaCO2. If hypoxemia persists and PaCO2 remains stable, the oxygen dose may be further increased until the target saturation is reached.

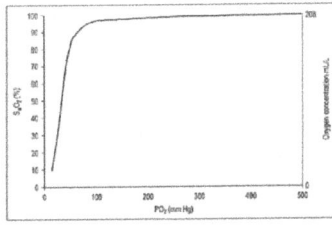

Figure 2-3 illustrates the hemoglobin-oxygen dissociation curve, which shows how oxygen binds to hemoglobin at varying levels of partial pressure.

Blood gas samples taken during the initial assessment, whether on room air or controlled oxygen, can provide valuable insight into the patient's condition. Venous blood samples can also be used for trend monitoring, provided consistency is maintained. A bicarbonate level above 30 mmol/L or an increase greater than 4 mmol/L per 1.3 kPa (10 mm Hg) rise in PaCO2 supports the diagnosis of chronic hypercapnia, assuming no other causes of metabolic alkalosis are present.

In cases where hypoxia persists or worsens, non-invasive positive-pressure ventilation (NIPPV) is a recommended option. Evidence supports its use in patients with worsening hypoxia, elevated $PaCO_2$, or declining consciousness. However, intubation should be considered a last resort. It is crucial not to abruptly withdraw supplemental oxygen in COPD patients, as this could lead to a catastrophic drop in PaO_2. Any reduction in oxygen therapy should be gradual, mirroring the approach used when increasing the dose.

In most cases, managing both hypoxia and hypercapnia can be achieved by titrating oxygen therapy. The underlying cause of ventilatory failure should be prioritized for treatment. Oxygen therapy, like any other medication, should be titrated to meet the patient's specific needs, ensuring the optimal dose is delivered.

Recent studies, including a randomized controlled trial

(RCT) comparing high-flow oxygen therapy (8 L/min) versus titrated oxygen therapy for patients with ST-segment elevation myocardial infarction, have raised concerns about the safety of uncontrolled oxygen administration. The trial found that uncontrolled oxygen use was associated with higher rates of arrhythmias, recurrent myocardial infarctions, and larger infarct sizes. These results suggest that oxygen should be considered a therapeutic agent, with its dose adjusted according to the patient's clinical needs. Similar studies on titrated oxygen therapy for asthma, pneumonia, and other conditions are ongoing, reinforcing the principle that oxygen should be managed like any other drug to provide the optimal dose for each patient.

Special oxygen delivery systems are also used in clinical settings, particularly in patients requiring prolonged oxygen therapy. Humidification is vital in these cases, especially for patients with endotracheal tubes or COPD with retained secretions. Oxygen humidification systems should deliver gas at 32°C to 36°C with high humidity (greater than 90%) to prevent airway dryness and irritation. These systems also provide additional benefits for treating hypothermic patients and addressing pulmonary complications from near-drowning.

Continuous positive airway pressure (CPAP) is another therapeutic option, particularly in cases of pulmonary edema, pneumonia, bronchiolitis, respiratory tract burns, and acute respiratory failure. CPAP improves oxygenation by increasing functional residual capacity and reducing pulmonary compliance, thus reducing intrapulmonary shunting and the work of breathing. CPAP is also associated with a reduction in the need for endotracheal intubation, though complications such as aspiration, barotrauma, and increased intracranial pressure may arise.

In some cases, hyperbaric oxygen therapy (HBO) is used to treat conditions like decompression illness, gas embolism, and carbon monoxide poisoning. HBO is delivered at pressures greater than 1 ATA, usually between 203 and 284 kPa, increasing the partial pressure of oxygen in the plasma. This enhanced oxygen delivery is beneficial when hemoglobin is non-functional, such as in carbon monoxide poisoning, and aids in the elimination of toxic gasses. HBO has demonstrated positive effects in managing ischemic tissues, promoting healing in chronic wounds, and treating anaerobic infections by targeting bacterial pathogens.

Oxygen therapy also carries potential risks, including equipment-related complications, carbon dioxide narcosis, and oxygen toxicity. Equipment-related issues can be prevented with proper monitoring and management of oxygen flow rates and circuit design. Carbon dioxide narcosis can be avoided by titrating oxygen therapy based on arterial blood gasses and conscious state, ensuring oxygen is never abruptly withdrawn, which could lead to severe hypoxia. Oxygen toxicity, particularly at high FIO2 levels, can lead to the formation of free radicals and damage to lung tissue, the central nervous system, and the eyes. Therefore, it is essential to monitor oxygen dosages carefully and adjust them to prevent prolonged exposure to high FIO2, which can lead to pulmonary fibrosis and other complications.

References

1. Cormack, R. S., & Lehane, J. (1984). Difficult intubation in obstetric patients. Anaesthesia, 39(11), 1105–1111.
2. Cook, T. M., Woodall, N., Harper, J., & Benger, J. (2011). Major airway management complications in the UK: Fourth National Audit Project results from the Royal College of Anaesthetists and the Difficult Airway Society.

British Journal of Anaesthesia, 106, 632–642.

3. Gerstein, N. S., Carey, M. C., Braude, D. A., et al. (2013). Effectiveness of facemask ventilation techniques among novice providers. Journal of Clinical Anesthesia, 25(3), 193–197.

4. Pracy, J. P., Brennan, L., Cook, T. M., et al. (2016). Surgical intervention during a "can't intubate, can't oxygenate" event: Emergency front-of-neck airway. Clinical Otolaryngology, 41(6), 624–626.

5. Chrimes, N. (2016). The vortex approach: A universal tool for high-acuity emergency airway management. British Journal of Anaesthesia, 117, i20–i27.

6. Petrucci, N., & De Feo, C. (2013). Lung protective ventilation strategies in acute respiratory distress syndrome: A systematic review. Cochrane Database of Systematic Reviews, 2, CD003844.

7. Alkhouri, H., Vassiliadis, J., Murray, M., et al. (2017). Emergency airway

management practices in Australian and New Zealand emergency departments: A multicenter descriptive study of 3710 intubations. Emergency Medicine Australasia, 29(5), 499–508.

Chapter 4
Haemodynamic Monitoring in the Emergency Department

Haemodynamics focuses on the physiology of blood flow and the forces within the circulatory system. Haemodynamic monitoring uses technology to assess these forces, helping clinicians make informed decisions in patient care. While basic monitoring is widely accepted, the notion that "not everything that counts can be counted" (Albert Einstein) is important, especially in the fast-paced environment of the emergency department (ED), where complex, costly monitoring systems may not be feasible.

Historical Context

Historically, only basic vital signs like temperature, pulse, and respirations were monitored until the early 20th century. Although tools for auscultatory blood pressure measurement were available, they only became widely used in the 1920s. The advent of intensive care and sophisticated haemodynamic techniques in the 1960s coincided with the electronic revolution. Despite advancements, evidence linking these technologies directly to improved patient outcomes remains scarce.

Practical Considerations in Haemodynamic Monitoring

Effective monitoring should be tailored to the clinical environment. For example, invasive procedures like Swan-Ganz catheter insertion, appropriate for intensive care units (ICUs), may be impractical or unsafe in a busy ED. Haemodynamic monitoring should only be used when it directly impacts clinical decision-making, as once irreversible damage occurs, further therapy is unlikely to be beneficial. Invasive monitoring carries risks, and protocols should be evidence-based to avoid worsening outcomes.

Key Principles for Effective Haemodynamic Monitoring

1. Clinical Relevance: Monitoring devices should measure variables that influence patient care.

2. Accuracy and Reproducibility: Data must be reliable and consistent.

3. Continuity: Continuous measurements are essential to track dynamic changes.

4. Clinical Utility: Data should guide treatment decisions.

5. Simplicity: Devices should be easy to operate and interpret.

6. Safety and Cost-Effectiveness: Technologies should be non-invasive or minimally invasive, with minimal risk to patients and within budgetary constraints.

Cardiovascular Physiology and Monitoring

The heart's ability to pump blood—cardiac output (CO)—is influenced by preload (blood volume), afterload (vascular resistance), and contractility. CO is typically measured indirectly, with tools estimating its value. Since CO reflects the metabolic needs of the body, accurate assessment is crucial, but routine CO measurements in patients with established diagnoses or those responding to initial treatment are generally not recommended.

Cardiac index (CI), which accounts for body surface area, is often preferred over CO alone as it provides a more accurate measure of tissue oxygen delivery. However, monitoring CO and CI remains controversial, especially in settings like the ED, where rapid decision-making is critical.

Haemodynamic Monitoring in the ED

In the ED, the role of haemodynamic monitoring remains uncertain, with various devices available but no universally accepted standard. Guidelines such as the Surviving Sepsis Campaign (2016) advocate for early, protocol-driven resuscitation, particularly for severe sepsis, to improve patient outcomes. However, the ED's limited capacity for intensive care presents challenges in applying these protocols.

Clinical Assessment vs. Technology

While advanced monitoring devices were developed due to limitations in clinical assessment, initial clinical evaluation—such as physical examination and vital signs—remains invaluable. In many cases, patients managed based on clinical judgment perform as well as those monitored with complex devices. The goal is to assess haemodynamics based on relevant clinical markers, like skin temperature, urine output, and mental status, which can help direct therapy more effectively.

Blood Pressure Monitoring and Clinical Endpoints

Blood pressure is a key measure in haemodynamic monitoring, with mean arterial pressure (MAP) providing a more reliable indicator of tissue perfusion than systolic or diastolic pressures. MAP is less affected by measurement techniques and is a better determinant of actual tissue blood flow.

In sepsis management, clinical endpoints such as urine output and skin temperature are critical markers of tissue perfusion and can guide early goal-directed therapy (EGDT). In heart failure, clinical signs of perfusion and congestion, such as orthopnea and jugular vein pulse, help identify the adequacy of cardiac output and guide therapeutic decisions.

Historically, low blood pressure was viewed as a primary indicator of shock and hemodynamic instability. However, this traditional approach is being reconsidered, as there is now a greater emphasis on global tissue hypoxia and the adequacy of cardiac output (CO). While Ohm's law suggests a relationship between mean arterial pressure (MAP) and CO, MAP is a regulated physiological variable, which means it may not reliably predict acute fluctuations in CO.

Non-Invasive Blood Pressure Measurement

Non-invasive blood pressure (NIBP) measurements, which began with the use of a sphygmomanometer and palpation in the late 1800s, were later enhanced by Korotkoff's auscultatory method in 1905. Initially, routine blood pressure assessments were not standard practice. Today, NIBP is the most common technique for initial cardiovascular evaluation in clinical settings, particularly in emergency departments (ED). Despite the differences between invasive and non-invasive measurements, NIBP remains a cornerstone of patient assessment and management.

Non-Invasive Blood Pressure Devices

NIBP techniques generally rely on assessing blood flow through the limbs. Automated oscillometric devices are now the standard for these measurements, while manual techniques (e.g., palpation or auscultation) are less commonly used in the ED. To ensure accurate results, the cuff width should be approximately 40% of the limb's mid-circumference. If the cuff size is inappropriate, it can result in erroneous readings. After inflation, the cuff pressure is gradually reduced while proprietary algorithms calculate systolic, diastolic, and mean arterial pressures. In normal pressure ranges, these measurements are accurate to within ±15 mm Hg, but in hypotensive and hypertensive states, oscillometric devices tend to overestimate and underestimate pressures, respectively. While complications are rare, repeated measurements can cause skin bruising, edema, or even ulceration.

Other Non-Invasive Monitoring Methods for Cardiac Output

Despite advances, a reliable non-invasive method to measure CO in the ED remains elusive. Existing devices do not consistently match the accuracy of invasive methods and may be too complex or time-consuming for use in the fast-paced ED environment.

Ultrasonic Cardiac Output Monitor (USCOM)

Introduced in 2001 in Australia, the USCOM uses continuous-wave Doppler ultrasound to non-invasively estimate CO. The device captures Doppler flow profiles either from the aortic or pulmonary window and calculates CO based on the velocity-time integral (VTI) and the target valve's cross-sectional area. USCOM offers quick and reliable CO estimates and can be particularly useful in initiating early goal-directed therapy (EGDT). Although studies show a good correlation with CO estimates from invasive methods like thermodilution via pulmonary artery catheter (PAC), the device's reliability may be affected by patient pathology and illness severity. Further research is needed to fully establish its role in ED practice. USCOM may be particularly helpful in monitoring changes in CO in response to treatment, such as fluid administration.

Oesophageal Doppler

Oesophageal Doppler monitoring (OD) uses a transducer positioned in the esophagus to measure CO via Doppler ultrasound. While transthoracic Doppler can struggle to provide acceptable flow signals, the transoesophageal method is more reliable. This technique requires minimal training and is becoming more feasible for bedside use by nursing staff. However, it is typically poorly tolerated by awake patients, limiting its use in the ED.

Transthoracic Echocardiography (TTE)

TTE is employed to assess left ventricular size, thickness, and function, as well as to determine the need for fluid administration. It is increasingly used in the ED as technology improves and more emergency physicians are trained in its application. TTE can guide treatment decisions by assessing left ventricular function, fluid responsiveness, and assessing the diameter and collapsibility of the inferior vena cava (IVC). However, the IVC collapsibility index, while useful in mechanically ventilated ICU patients, has limited value in spontaneously breathing patients and is influenced by factors such as left and right ventricular function and pulmonary hypertension.

Invasive Blood Pressure Monitoring

Arterial cannulation allows for continuous blood pressure measurement and beat-to-beat waveform display. The procedure involves inserting a cannula into an artery, connecting it to a pressure transducer, and zeroing the system to the phlebostatic axis. Radial artery cannulation is preferred due to its accessibility and low complication rate. However, other sites, such as femoral and axillary arteries, are used when necessary. The main risks of arterial cannulation include hematoma formation, bleeding, and potential nerve injury.

Use of Invasive Blood Pressure Monitoring

Invasive blood pressure monitoring is crucial for all hemodynamically unstable patients, especially those receiving vasopressors or vasodilators. Relying solely on NIBP monitoring may not provide sufficient diagnostic information, particularly in cases of sepsis. Additional methods of hemodynamic monitoring, such as invasive devices, should be considered for these patients.

Central Venous Pressure Monitoring

Central venous pressure (CVP) monitoring, which has been in use since the 1920s, was initially instrumental in assessing right heart function and intravascular volume. However, its correlation with left heart function in critically ill patients is unreliable. CVP is now considered a rough estimate of right atrial pressure (RAP), with its usefulness dependent on dynamic changes rather than absolute values.

Central Venous Access

Central venous access is achieved by inserting a catheter

into a peripheral or central vein. The catheter tip is positioned at the junction of the superior vena cava and right atrium. Common insertion sites include the internal jugular, subclavian, and femoral veins, with site selection influenced by the patient's anatomy and clinical condition.

Indications for Central Venous Access

Indications for central venous access include fluid and electrolyte replacement, drug administration (e.g., vasopressors), monitoring CVP, sampling central venous blood to assess oxygen saturation, and the insertion of more invasive devices such as PACs.

Complications of Central Venous Access

Complications can be categorized as early and late. Early complications include pneumothorax, hematothorax, dysrhythmias, and injury to surrounding structures. Late complications include catheter-related sepsis, erosion of the superior vena cava, and venous thrombosis.

Central Venous Oxygen Saturation

Central venous oxygen saturation (ScvO2) is measured from blood obtained via the central venous catheter and reflects the balance between oxygen delivery and consumption. In healthy individuals, oxygen extraction is around 25-30%, and an ScvO2 greater than 65% indicates an optimal balance. ScvO2 levels below 70% are associated with higher complication rates and longer hospital stays in postoperative ICU patients. Continuous monitoring of ScvO2 is valuable in guiding treatment and ensuring effective oxygenation.

Transpulmonary Thermodilution for Hemodynamic Monitoring

Transpulmonary thermodilution is a technique used to assess hemodynamics by measuring preload and volume responsiveness through global end-diastolic blood volume (GEDV) and intrathoracic blood volume (ITBV).

Additionally, it provides insights into the amount of extravascular lung water (EVLW), which reflects the water content outside the pulmonary vasculature, including the interstitial and alveolar spaces, making it a useful marker for pulmonary edema. This method is considered accurate and comparable to pulmonary artery thermodilution.

The PiCCO system, which utilizes this technique, continuously monitors critical parameters, including:

PiCCO
Arterial blood pressure
Heart rate (HR)
Stroke volume (SV)
Systemic vascular resistance (SVR)
ITBV
EVLW
Cardiac function index (CFI)
Clinical Use of Parameters
ITBV: This is indicative of cardiac preload and aids in fluid management. Its clinical utility aligns closely with GEDV, particularly when dynamic volume responsiveness

measures like stroke volume variation (SVV) and systolic pressure variation (SPV) are not applicable.

EVLW: Correlating with the extravascular thermal volume in the lungs, EVLW is a key parameter in assessing and managing fluid balance, especially in patients with existing pulmonary edema.

CFI: This index, calculated as the ratio of cardiac output (CO) to GEDV, reflects the heart's contractility, providing a preload-independent measurement of the heart's inotropic state. Though potentially valuable in assessing cardiac performance, its added benefit compared to the individual components (CO and GEDV) remains uncertain.

Advantages of the PiCCO System

The PiCCO system is advantageous in its less invasive approach compared to a pulmonary artery catheter (PAC), requiring only a central venous catheter and an arterial line, both of which are commonly used in critically ill patients. This minimizes the risk of complications associated with more invasive monitoring techniques. Moreover, PiCCO provides comprehensive data that can help guide hemodynamic management with reliable parameters. However, its use may be limited in cases with restricted femoral artery access, intracardiac shunts, aortic anomalies, or during extracorporeal circulation.

Limitations of the PiCCO System

Despite its advantages, there are contraindications to the PiCCO system, including:

Difficulty obtaining femoral artery access (e.g., in burn patients)

Inaccurate measurements in the presence of intracardiac shunts, aortic aneurysms, aortic stenosis, or after pneumonectomy

Potential measurement errors in cases of rapidly changing body temperature or during extracorporeal circulation

Drift in values following significant changes in vascular compliance

Pulmonary Artery Catheter (PAC) and Its Declining Role

Historically considered the gold standard for monitoring unstable circulation, the PAC (Swan-Ganz catheter) has fallen out of favor, with studies indicating that its use does not improve patient outcomes and may even worsen them. The insertion of a PAC is technically demanding and associated with significant risks, including hematoma, infection, pulmonary infarction, and arrhythmias. As a result, current guidelines discourage routine use of PACs, particularly in emergency settings.

Conclusion and Future Developments

In emergency medicine, the challenge lies in selecting the most appropriate hemodynamic monitoring methods that can improve both diagnosis and management. A stepwise approach, starting with clinical assessment and escalating monitoring based on the patient's condition, is currently recommended.

Future advancements in monitoring technologies show promise, particularly in the assessment of microcirculation and metabolic status. Techniques such as near-infrared spectroscopy (NIRS) and NADPH fluorescence microscopy are being explored for real-time cellular assessment, especially in cases of shock. NIRS, in particular, has gained attention for its non-invasive ability to measure peripheral tissue oxygenation, and its role in conditions like trauma, cardiac failure, and sepsis is being further validated. Other promising developments include microcirculation assessment via videomicroscopy and non-invasive tonometry to reconstruct central aortic pressures.

In conclusion, while technologies like PiCCO are already showing significant potential, continued research and technological improvements will be crucial to optimizing their use in clinical practice.

References

1. Boldrini, R., Fasano, L., & Nava, S. (2012). Insights into the use of noninvasive mechanical ventilation. Current Opinion in Critical Care, 18, 48–53.

2. Groombridge, C., Chin, C. W., Hanrahan, B., & Holdgate, A. (2016). Evaluation of preoxygenation techniques in settings outside the operating room. Academic Emergency Medicine, 23(3), 342–346.

3. Ramachandran, S. K., Cosnowski, A., Shanks, A., & Turner, C. R. (2010). The impact of nasal oxygen delivery on apneic oxygenation during extended laryngoscopy in obese patients: A randomized controlled trial. Journal of Clinical Anesthesia, 22(3), 164–168.

4. Benumof, J. L., Dagg, R., & Benumof, R. (1997). Analysis of critical hemoglobin desaturation prior to recovery from paralysis after succinylcholine administration

at a dose of 1 mg/kg. Anesthesiology, 87(4), 979–982.

5. Weingart, S. D., Trueger, N. S., Wong, N., et al. (2015). A prospective study on delayed sequence intubation for emergency airway management. Annals of Emergency Medicine, 65(4), 349–355.

6. Bhatia, N., Bhagat, H., & Sen, I. (2014). Current perspectives on the role of cricoid pressure in airway management. Journal of Anaesthesiology Clinical Pharmacology, 30(1), 3–6.

7. Gerstein, N. S., Carey, M. C., Braude, D. A., et al. (2013). A comparative study on facemask ventilation techniques by novice practitioners. Journal of Clinical Anesthesia, 25(3), 193–197.

8. Chrimes, N. (2016). The Vortex approach: A comprehensive tool for managing emergency airways in critical situations. British Journal of Anaesthesia, 117, i20–i27.

9. Petrucci, N., & De Feo, C. (2013). Strategies for lung-protective ventilation in acute respiratory distress syndrome: Evidence from a Cochrane review. Cochrane Database of Systematic Reviews, (2), CD003844.

10. Alkhouri, H., Vassiliadis, J., Murray, M., et al. (2017). Emergency airway management practices in Australian and New Zealand emergency departments: A multicenter study of 3,710 intubations. Emergency Medicine Australasia, 29(5), 499–508.

Chapter 5
Shock Overview

Shock is a critical clinical syndrome where inadequate tissue perfusion leads to insufficient oxygen supply, impairing cellular and organ function. In the early stages, the effects of insufficient perfusion can be reversed, but prolonged oxygen deprivation leads to widespread cellular hypoxia, disrupting essential biochemical processes. This results in cellular damage, including membrane ion pump dysfunction, impaired intracellular pH regulation, cellular edema, and ultimately cell death.

Shock is traditionally classified based on its underlying cause, with management typically aimed at addressing immediate cardiorespiratory abnormalities and adjusting the diagnosis based on response to treatment. However, the primary focus is often on stabilizing vital functions, with the underlying cause addressed later. Recognizing shock can be challenging, especially in vulnerable populations like the very young or elderly. Pre-existing medical conditions and medication use can alter the body's compensatory mechanisms, complicating the diagnosis. In any emergency where symptoms, signs, or lab findings suggest abnormal organ function, clinicians must consider the possibility of shock. Early, targeted treatment has been shown to improve patient outcomes.

Aetiology and Epidemiology

Shock arises from dysfunction within the cardiovascular system, often with multiple contributing factors. If the cause is known, shock is categorized based on the mechanism—such as hypovolaemic, cardiogenic, septic, neurogenic, or anaphylactic shock—each guiding specific therapeutic interventions.

When the cause is unclear or the response to treatment is inadequate, the following physiological classifications help in decision-making:

Hypovolaemia: Reduced preload due to either intravascular or extravascular fluid loss (e.g., trauma, gastrointestinal bleeding, burns, or ascites).

Distributive shock: Reduced total peripheral resistance, typically due to arterial vasodilation or altered venous capacitance (e.g., sepsis, anaphylaxis, neurogenic shock).

Obstructive shock: Impaired heart filling due to external factors such as tension pneumothorax, pericardial tamponade, or large pulmonary embolism.

Cardiogenic shock: Pump dysfunction, which can arise from systolic or diastolic dysfunction, arrhythmias, or valvular problems.

Essentials of Shock Management

1. Shock is categorized into disturbances in intravascular volume, vascular resistance, cardiac filling, and myocardial pumping, with multiple overlapping causes often present.

2. Hypotension is a significant sign of shock, but it may not appear until late in the disease course.

3. All shock patients should be evaluated for hypovolaemia, with early volume resuscitation being a primary concern.

4. Initial interventions target the physiological deficit, acting as a test of the working diagnosis, with continuous reassessment guiding further treatment.

5. Common management errors include delayed diagnosis,

insufficient fluid resuscitation, inadequate control of the underlying issue, delayed ventilatory support, and overreliance on inappropriate treatments.

6. Cardiogenic shock outcomes improve with revascularization and surgical interventions, but the benefits of thrombolysis and intra-aortic balloon counterpulsation remain unproven.

7. In septic shock, evidence supports fluid resuscitation, vasopressors, timely antibiotics, and source control over adjunctive therapies.

Pathophysiology

Organs can autoregulate blood flow based on metabolic demands, provided perfusion is adequate. This balance depends on the mean arterial pressure (MAP), which is influenced by cardiac output (CO) and total peripheral resistance (TPR). A decrease in CO or TPR leads to a reduction in MAP, disrupting organ perfusion. CO is determined by stroke volume (SV) and heart rate (HR), and preload affects SV, which in turn impacts CO. In shock, factors like reduced venous tone, endothelial damage, and heart dysfunction contribute to the failure of adequate perfusion.

Compensatory Mechanisms

In response to shock, the body activates neurohormonal mechanisms, increasing catecholamines, angiotensin, aldosterone, and vasopressin levels. This results in symptoms such as tachycardia, anxiety, thirst, reduced urinary output, and skin blood flow diversion. Although blood flow to vital organs such as the brain and heart is preserved, peripheral organs suffer. Fluid shifts from the interstitium to the intravascular compartment may temporarily mask the effects of volume loss.

Decompensated Shock

If shock persists without adequate treatment, the body fails to regenerate ATP, impairing cellular function. This leads to myocardial dysfunction (both systolic and diastolic) and vascular failure, even in the presence of high circulating catecholamines. This stage is known as decompensated shock, where tissue perfusion cannot be restored by compensatory mechanisms alone.

Clinical Features

Initial clinical signs of shock stem from inadequate tissue perfusion and multi-organ dysfunction. Key indicators include:

Mental state: Decreased cerebral perfusion manifests as confusion, anxiety, or even coma.

Symptoms: Patients often report thirst, cold extremities, or a sense of impending doom, along with presyncopal symptoms like nausea.

Peripheral circulation: Vasoconstriction leads to cold, pale, or mottled skin, and delayed capillary refill (more than 4 seconds) is observed. In some cases (e.g., sepsis), skin may be warm due to vasodilation.

Hypotension: Defined as a systolic BP less than 90 mm Hg or a drop of more than 30 mm Hg from baseline. A low BP is a late finding in shock, with mean arterial pressure (MAP) now considered a more accurate indicator.

Tachycardia: Frequently present but can be masked by medications or aging. Bradycardia may occur in specific scenarios like inferior myocardial infarction.

Tachypnoea: A sensitive but non-specific predictor of deterioration in shock.

Core temperature: Can be low, normal, or elevated, influenced by various factors such as age and underlying conditions.

Oliguria: Reduced urine output is commonly observed.

Initial Management

Effective shock management follows structured protocols like those from the Advanced Trauma Life Support (ATLS) or Advanced Cardiac Life Support (ACLS) guidelines. These frameworks promote systematic assessment and therapy, with treatments adjusted based on clinical responses and diagnostic findings. Urgent escalation to a multidisciplinary team and reassessment of patient status are critical, as shock represents a high risk of mortality.

Echocardiogram and Ultrasound Use in Resuscitation

Incorporating echocardiography (TTE) into resuscitation algorithms has become standard practice when available. The Focused Assessment with Sonography for Trauma (FAST) is commonly used to identify free abdominal fluid and exclude conditions such as pericardial tamponade. Advanced ultrasound technology allows for comprehensive evaluations, including detection of intrathoracic free fluid, measurement of aortic or vena cava diameters, and assessment of cardiac function. This includes examining ventricular cavity dimensions (to assess adequate filling), ejection fraction, regional wall motion abnormalities (which may indicate ischemia), and potential valvular dysfunction.

Invasive Monitoring in the Emergency Department

Invasive monitoring in the emergency department (ED) provides real-time data crucial for guiding resuscitation:

Intra-arterial blood pressure (BP) monitoring provides more accurate and timely detection of hypotension compared to intermittent non-invasive methods.

Systolic pressure variation (SVV) and pulse pressure variation (PPV) during mechanical ventilation are reliable indicators of fluid responsiveness and can be used as alternatives to central venous pressure (CVP) and pulmonary artery wedge pressure.

Central venous pressure (CVP) trends are followed post-fluid administration to assess volume responsiveness.

End-tidal CO_2 in ventilated patients, compared with arterial $PaCO_2$, may highlight inadequate lung perfusion and guide resuscitation efforts.

Central venous oxygen saturation ($ScvO_2$) measured through a central venous catheter can indicate oxygen delivery and consumption balance. ScvO2 levels below 65%-75% suggest a mismatch between oxygen delivery and consumption.

Pulse contour analysis devices (e.g., Flowtrac) utilize arterial waveform analysis to provide cardiac output (CO) and other derived parameters, assisting in the management of resuscitation.

Advanced monitoring such as pulmonary artery catheterization, PiCCO (peripheral invasive cardiac output monitors), and transesophageal echocardiography (TOE) are typically reserved for intensive care settings.

Goal-Directed Resuscitation

Goal-directed resuscitation involves adjusting various interventions (e.g., fluid volume, inotropes, vasopressors) to achieve predefined cardiac output (CO) levels. Early studies proposed that targeting supranormal CO and oxygen delivery could improve outcomes, but subsequent large-scale randomized controlled trials

(RCTs) failed to confirm these findings. Notably, the Rivers trial in 2001 suggested improved survival in septic shock through a resuscitation protocol guided by CVP, mean arterial pressure (MAP), and central venous oxygen saturation. However, subsequent trials showed inconsistent benefits, particularly in trauma patients, and often involved increased fluid administration. Clear clinical goals are crucial for coordinating efforts during resuscitation but should be customized to each patient's needs.

Fluid Therapy in Shock Management

Fluid Selection

The general approach to fluid resuscitation follows the principle of replacing fluids lost at the rate they are lost. While there is no consensus on the superiority of any specific fluid type in shock, 0.9% normal saline remains the most common choice. Evidence suggests that hypotonic or glucose-containing fluids can be harmful in critically ill patients. Balanced solutions, such as Hartmann's solution, may reduce the risk of hyperchloremic acidosis compared to saline, though clinical relevance remains uncertain. The SAFE study found no significant difference in outcomes between saline and human albumin solution. Additionally, hydroxyethyl starch is not superior to saline and is associated with more complications. In cases of significant blood loss or dilution, maintaining oxygen-carrying capacity and coagulation is crucial, with blood transfusion triggers often set at hemoglobin levels between 70-90 g/L.

Fluid Administration

Fluid is typically administered in boluses ranging from 10 to 40 mL/kg, with a preferred average of 20 mL/kg. If the heart's compliance is compromised or if it is already "full," a smaller bolus may be given, with close monitoring of the clinical response. Flow rates are achieved using large-bore cannulas (16-20 gauge), and in urgent cases, gravity-driven infusion or pressure bags may be used.

Fluid Administration Routes

Fluid can be delivered through central lines, peripheral intravenous catheters, or intraosseous needles. Ultrasound-guided access is considered in challenging cases, and central lines or PICC (peripherally inserted central catheters) lines may be necessary for continuous vasopressor/inotropic infusion.

Complications of Fluid Therapy

Several complications may arise from aggressive fluid therapy:

Hypothermia can occur with large-volume infusions, necessitating warmed fluids and active warming devices.

Coagulopathy may develop from dilution, sepsis, hypothermia, or acidosis, with fresh frozen plasma (FFP) used to address dilutional causes.

Pulmonary and tissue edema may occur, often linked to the inflammatory response in shock, with management through ventilation or diuresis if required.

Anaphylaxis to colloids or blood products is rare but may complicate resuscitation.

Inotropes and Vasopressors in Shock Management

Choice of Inotrope/Vasopressor

Vasopressors and inotropes are both essential in managing shock, but their effects overlap significantly. Vasopressors increase vascular tone, raising mean arterial pressure (MAP) and improving preload, while inotropes enhance myocardial contractility, potentially improving cardiac output (CO) and BP. The choice of medication depends on the clinical scenario, institutional preferences, and known side effects. For instance:

Dopamine is often less preferred due to an increased risk of arrhythmias and lack of renal protective effects.

Dobutamine can improve contractility but may drop BP, requiring careful use in hypotensive patients.

Levosimendan and dopexamine have limited use due to insufficient evidence supporting their efficacy.

Administration and Titration

Vasopressors/inotropes are typically administered through central lines using precise infusion protocols. Titration of these drugs should aim to achieve the desired BP or perfusion goals. Inotropes or vasopressors should be used only after adequate preload is established, as their use without proper fluid resuscitation can worsen outcomes.

Absolute Hypovolemia

Clinical Features:

Shock due to absolute hypovolemia often results from fluid loss, which could be from the vascular system, gastrointestinal tract, kidneys, or through evaporation. A thorough history and clinical examination can help identify the source of fluid loss. Bleeding should always be considered and ruled out in all cases of hypovolemia. Common signs include evidence of decreased preload, such as flat neck veins, a consequence of low central venous pressure (CVP).

Relevant Investigations:

If bleeding is suspected, surgical intervention is often the most effective first step to stop the bleeding and may occur alongside resuscitation efforts. If the initial resuscitation stabilizes the patient, further imaging studies such as ultrasound or CT with contrast angiography can help locate the site of hemorrhage. In cases of severe pelvic trauma, angiographic embolization can be a lifesaving intervention.

Therapy:

Initial Resuscitation: Begin fluid resuscitation as previously outlined, ensuring that the patient is kept warm to prevent hypothermia.

Positioning: Passive leg elevation has been shown to be more effective than the Trendelenburg position in increasing left ventricular end-diastolic volume, stroke volume (SV), and cardiac output (CO), although these effects are temporary.

Hemorrhage Control: External bleeding should be controlled with firm, direct manual pressure. Tourniquets, while associated with some risks, may be beneficial in the short term for controlling limb hemorrhage.

Surgical Consultation: A prompt surgical consultation is essential, particularly when dealing with trauma that involves significant blood loss. Efforts to normalize the systolic blood pressure (SBP) in trauma patients with bleeding may be harmful, especially in cases of penetrating abdominal trauma. For these patients, a minimal-volume fluid resuscitation approach is recommended until surgical intervention can be performed. This minimal-volume approach involves administering small boluses (250 mL) or fluids to maintain peripheral perfusion and cerebral and myocardial oxygenation.

Fluid Resuscitation: In major hemorrhagic shock, packed red

blood cells (PRBC) are indicated if oxygen delivery is impaired, or hemoglobin (Hb) levels fall below 70 g/L. If coagulopathy is suspected, fresh frozen plasma (FFP) and platelets should be given as part of a major transfusion protocol. For patients with non-hemorrhagic hypovolemic shock or those with minor blood loss, warmed crystalloid solutions are usually sufficient.

Hypertonic Saline: Hypertonic saline (3% or 7%) has been explored as an option in traumatic brain injury (TBI) but remains unproven. Despite this, it is often the initial fluid of choice in hemorrhaging patients, particularly in military settings.

Blood Substitutes: Currently, there are no conclusive recommendations for the use of blood substitutes like modified hemoglobin or perfluorocarbon-based products.

Preload and Contractility Considerations: Conditions such as tension pneumothorax, cardiac tamponade, and myocardial contusion must also be considered in the hypovolemic trauma patient. Bedside ultrasound is essential to detect these conditions, and increasing preload remains beneficial in these settings.

Relative Hypovolemia

Relative hypovolemia can result from conditions like anaphylaxis, Addisonian crisis, neurogenic shock, septic shock, or drug/toxin effects.

Anaphylaxis:

The primary treatment for anaphylactic shock involves the administration of epinephrine (adrenaline), along with supplemental oxygen and fluids. The patient should be positioned supine with legs elevated.

Adrenal Shock:

Hypotension due to adrenal insufficiency is rare but should be suspected in patients with a history of steroid use or in those presenting with hypotension, polyuria, and relatively high urinary sodium levels (e.g., >20 mmol/L).

Neurogenic Shock:

Neurogenic shock is characterized by hypotension, bradycardia, and hypothermia, typically occurring after acute spinal cord injury due to the loss of sympathetic tone. About 25% of patients with complete cervical cord injuries may require hemodynamic support. Other causes of hypovolemia or shock, such as bleeding or cardiac tamponade, should still be actively investigated.

Septic Shock:

Septic shock is defined as sepsis associated with hypotension and/or poor perfusion. Despite rapid fluid resuscitation, persistent hypotension or signs of organ hypoperfusion indicate the need for vasopressor or inotropic support. Vasopressin, administered at 0.04 U/min, has shown no survival advantage in septic shock. Studies suggest albumin may offer survival benefits, and hydrocortisone may help in shock resistance to other treatments. However, these treatments have shown no definitive impact on mortality (see Chapter 2.5).

Drug Effects:

Certain drugs or toxins can cause hypotension by interfering with vascular tone or cardiac contractility. Managing these cases involves fluid administration or the use of inotropes and pressors. If the drug affects vasopressor or ionotropic receptors, physiological antagonism or stimulation of alternative receptors may counteract the drug's effects.

Cardiac Causes of Shock: Cardiogenic Shock

Cardiogenic shock occurs when the heart cannot provide sufficient blood to meet the body's metabolic demands. It is clinically defined by a systolic blood pressure (SBP) of less than 90 mm Hg or a mean arterial pressure (MAP) more than 30 mm Hg below baseline for at least 30 minutes. In severe cases, a significant arterio-venous oxygen difference, along with a cardiac index of less than 2.2 L/min/m^2 and elevated pulmonary capillary wedge pressure (>15 mm Hg), may be observed.

Cardiogenic shock is diagnosed when the patient fails to improve with correction of hypoxemia, hypovolemia, arrhythmias, and acidosis. Signs of inadequate tissue perfusion include oliguria, cyanosis, and altered mental status.

Etiology:

The most common cause of cardiogenic shock is acute myocardial infarction (MI), which complicates 5-8% of MI cases and has a mortality rate of 56-74%. Cardiogenic shock is the leading cause of death in the hospital following a heart attack. Other causes include valvular rupture, critical stenosis, septal or free wall rupture, and atrial myxoma. Obstructive causes such as cardiac tamponade or pulmonary embolism are typically distinguished from cardiogenic shock due to the absence of myocardial dysfunction.

Older patients, those with diabetes, or individuals with previous myocardial infarctions are at higher risk of cardiogenic shock, particularly if they have multivessel disease. The highest risk is seen in patients with left main coronary artery involvement. Aggressive revascularization within 12 hours of symptom onset improves survival.

Pathophysiology:

Cardiogenic shock is associated with increased myocardial oxygen demand, which exacerbates ischemia and reduces contractility, stroke volume, and cardiac output. This creates a vicious cycle of further damage. Pulmonary edema worsens hypoxia and hypoperfusion, while vascular redistribution leads to organ failure and metabolic acidosis.

Clinical Features:

In addition to previously mentioned signs of shock, cardiogenic shock presents with symptoms of excessive catecholamine release such as tachycardia, pallor, poor capillary refill, and signs of low cardiac output like reduced urine output and elevated lactate levels. Blood pressure may initially remain within normal limits due to compensatory mechanisms. Pulmonary edema may be evidenced by crackles and the presence of a third heart sound gallop rhythm, indicating reduced ventricular compliance. In right heart failure (secondary to left heart failure or right ventricular infarction), elevated jugular venous pressure (JVP), hepatic congestion, and peripheral edema may be present.

Investigations:

ECG: A 12-lead ECG can help identify ischemic territories and guide the need for reperfusion therapy. Additional leads (V4R and V7–9) should be used to rule out right-sided or posterior MI.

Troponin levels: Elevated troponin I or T levels help confirm myocardial injury.

Chest X-ray: Pulmonary edema and cardiac enlargement may be evident.

TTE (Transthoracic Echocardiography): Should be performed to evaluate myocardial function and exclude conditions such as cardiac tamponade.

TOE (Transesophageal Echocardiography): In cases of undiagnosed shock, TOE can identify loculated pericardial effusion, pulmonary embolism, or valvular lesions.

Emergency Department Therapy:

Management begins with initial care and monitoring, including myocardial infarction management according to local protocols. If cardiogenic shock is identified, a discussion with a referral center for potential revascularization is critical. Intubation may be necessary for respiratory support, and invasive blood pressure monitoring is recommended. Arrhythmias contributing to shock should be managed according to ACLS guidelines. Hypovolemia should always be corrected by administering small fluid boluses (250 mL) and reassessing the patient's response. Preload should be carefully managed, particularly in patients with right ventricular involvement, as in inferior MI. Monitoring should focus on signs of improved perfusion, such as urine output and lactate normalization. If shock persists despite appropriate fluid resuscitation, urgent revascularization or mechanical support, such as an intra-aortic balloon pump, may be required.

Sepsis and septic shock

Sepsis is a leading global cause of preventable death, with over 30 million cases each year and responsible for more than 5 million deaths annually. Septic shock, a severe form of sepsis marked by significant circulatory dysfunction, drastically increases mortality rates. The global variation in septic shock mortality is notable, with figures ranging from 39.3% in the United States to 65.2% in India, and a much lower 22.0% in Australia and New Zealand for ICU-admitted septic patients. Over the past decade, the incidence of sepsis has continued to rise, emphasizing the importance of prompt intervention, particularly in emergency settings, where early management has been shown to improve patient outcomes.

Aetiology and Pathophysiology

Sepsis is predominantly caused by bacterial infections, although the distribution of responsible pathogens has evolved. A study involving 14,000 ICU patients from 75 countries showed that 70% of infected individuals had microbial isolates, with 62% being gram-negative bacteria (20% Pseudomonas spp., 16% Escherichia coli) and 47% gram-positive bacteria (20% Staphylococcus aureus). Fungal infections accounted for 19% of cases. The most common infection sites include the lungs (64%), abdomen (20%), bloodstream (15%), and urinary tract (14%).

The pathogenesis of sepsis involves complex interactions between the host and the pathogen. Proinflammatory and anti-inflammatory responses are triggered by pattern-recognition receptors, such as Toll-like receptors and nucleotide-binding oligomerization domain-like receptors. These responses lead to the activation of neutrophils, endothelial injury, increased vascular permeability, and the release of nitric oxide (NO), resulting in vasodilation. Coagulation abnormalities, including an increase in procoagulants and a decrease in anticoagulants, further contribute to the condition's severity, leading to reduced vascular resistance, tissue hypoperfusion, organ dysfunction, and septic shock.

Definitions

In 2016, the Sepsis-3 Task Force defined sepsis as life-threatening organ dysfunction due to a dysregulated host response to infection, identifiable by an acute increase of ≥ 2 points in the Sequential Organ Failure Assessment (SOFA) score. Septic shock is a more severe subset of sepsis, characterized by profound circulatory and metabolic abnormalities that significantly increase mortality. The use of the Systemic Inflammatory Response

Syndrome (SIRS) criteria for diagnosing sepsis and the term "severe sepsis" have been excluded from the Sepsis-3 definitions.

Screening

The quick SOFA (qSOFA) tool is recommended for identifying adults with suspected infections who are at high risk for poor outcomes. The presence of two or more of the following qSOFA criteria suggests possible sepsis: (1) respiratory rate ≥22/min, (2) Glasgow Coma Scale (GCS) <15, and (3) systolic blood pressure ≤100 mm Hg. Septic shock is identified when sepsis is present with both of the following: (1) persistent hypotension requiring vasopressors to maintain a mean arterial pressure (MAP) ≥65 mm Hg, and (2) a serum lactate level >2 mmol/L despite adequate volume resuscitation.

Although the Sepsis-3 guidelines exclude SIRS criteria, modified SIRS may still be helpful in detecting infection, particularly in cases where organ dysfunction is not yet evident. The criteria include abnormal temperature (≥38.3°C or <36.0°C), heart rate >90 bpm, respiratory rate >20/min, altered mental status, abnormal white blood cell count, and elevated blood glucose.

History and Examination

Diagnosing sepsis can be challenging due to its often non-specific and vague symptoms. Key indicators include fever, tachycardia, respiratory distress, altered mental state, and hypotension. A thorough examination should assess vital signs and identify risk factors such as recent infections, surgery, or invasive procedures. Early signs of sepsis may include mild tachycardia and fever, which can progress to shock, altered mental status, cyanosis, and oliguria as the condition worsens.

Management

Sepsis and septic shock require immediate medical intervention. The Surviving Sepsis Campaign (SSC) guidelines emphasize the need for rapid treatment, including early antibiotic administration and fluid resuscitation. The updated "Hour-1 Bundle" includes the following elements:

Measure lactate levels to assess tissue perfusion. If the initial lactate level is >2 mmol/L, it should be rechecked in 2 to 4 hours.

Obtain blood cultures before starting antibiotics to help identify the pathogen, but do not delay antibiotic administration.

Administer broad-spectrum intravenous antibiotics to cover likely pathogens. Once the pathogen is identified, antibiotics can be narrowed based on susceptibility testing.

Initiate fluid resuscitation with 30 mL/kg of intravenous crystalloid for hypotension or elevated lactate. This should be completed within 3 hours of sepsis recognition.

If hypotension persists after fluid resuscitation, apply vasopressors to achieve a MAP ≥65 mm Hg, with norepinephrine as the first-choice agent.

Societal and Governmental Guidelines

Various national and international bodies, including the UK Sepsis Trust, the Royal College of Emergency Medicine, and the Clinical Excellence Commission in New South Wales, have developed guidelines and quality-improvement initiatives aimed at improving sepsis outcomes. These include protocols for early recognition, resuscitation with IV fluids and antibiotics, and referral to senior clinicians. The "Sepsis Kills!" a program in New South Wales, for example, showed an increase in the percentage of patients receiving antibiotics within 60 minutes and a reduction in sepsis-related mortality.

Early Goal-Directed Therapy

The concept of Early Goal-Directed Therapy (EGDT) was introduced in 2001, suggesting that targeted physiological interventions could reduce mortality by optimizing tissue oxygenation. However, more recent randomized controlled trials (ProCESS, ARISE, ProMISe) have not demonstrated a significant benefit of EGDT over usual resuscitation protocols. These trials suggest that while EGDT may be effective in certain settings, the outcomes may not be significantly different when compared to standard care approaches for sepsis management.

Empirical Initial Intravenous Antibiotic Recommendations for Severe Sepsis

In patients with severe sepsis, antibiotic treatment is chosen based on the likely source of infection. The recommendations are as follows:

1. Unknown Source of Infection:

The first-line treatment includes Flucloxacillin 2 g every 4 hours, along with Gentamicin 7 mg/kg (ideal body weight) daily. The doses of Gentamicin are adjusted based on the patient's creatinine levels.

If there is a risk of methicillin-resistant Staphylococcus aureus (MRSA), add Vancomycin 25–

30 mg/kg as a loading dose, adjusted for creatinine levels.

If the patient has mild penicillin hypersensitivity, substitute Flucloxacillin with Cefazolin 2 g every 6 hours.

For immediate penicillin hypersensitivity, administer Vancomycin (as described above) and Gentamicin (as described above).

2. Biliary/Gastrointestinal Infection:

Treat with Amoxicillin or Ampicillin 2 g every 6 hours, or substitute with Ceftriaxone 1 g every 12 hours for patients with mild penicillin hypersensitivity (omit for immediate hypersensitivity).

Add Gentamicin 7 mg/kg daily, with dose adjustments based on creatinine levels.

In cases with chronic biliary obstruction, include Metronidazole 500 mg IV every 12 hours.

3. Community-Acquired Pneumonia:

The regimen includes Azithromycin 500 mg daily, combined with Ceftriaxone 1 g every 12 hours.

Alternatively, use Benzylpenicillin 1.2 g every 4 hours with Gentamicin 7 mg/kg daily and Azithromycin 500 mg daily.

In severe cases of immediate penicillin hypersensitivity, use Moxifloxacin 400 mg daily.

4. Hospital-Acquired Pneumonia:

Treat with Piperacillin + Tazobactam 4+0.5 g every 6 hours, along with Vancomycin 25–30 mg/kg as a loading dose, adjusted according to creatinine levels.

5. Urinary Tract Infection:

Start with Amoxicillin or Ampicillin 2 g every 6 hours, omitting the drug in cases of immediate penicillin hypersensitivity, and include Gentamicin 7 mg/kg daily (with dose adjustments based on creatinine).

If extended-spectrum beta-lactamase (ESBL)-producing organisms are suspected, use Amikacin 16–20 mg/kg daily or Meropenem 1 g every 8 hours.

6. Cellulitis:

The standard treatment is Flucloxacillin 2 g every 6 hours.

If there is a risk of MRSA, add Vancomycin 25–30 mg/kg as a loading dose, adjusted based on creatinine.

If Gram-negative organisms are suspected, add Gentamicin 7 mg/kg daily.

7. Neurological Infections (including Meningitis):

Begin with Dexamethasone 10 mg, administered with or just before the first dose of antibiotics, continuing every 6 hours for 4 days.

Use Ceftriaxone 4 g daily or 2 g every 12 hours, reviewed within 48 hours.

If Listeria infection is suspected, add Benzylpenicillin 2.4 g every 4 hours.

In cases of immediate penicillin hypersensitivity, use Vancomycin 25–30 mg/kg (loading dose), Ciprofloxacin 400 mg every 8 hours, and if Listeria is a concern, add Trimethoprim + Sulfamethoxazole 160 mg + 800 mg every 6 hours.

Renal Replacement Therapy in Sepsis

Septic shock can lead to circulatory dysfunction and acute kidney injury. Continuous renal replacement therapy (CRRT) is recommended for patients with fluid imbalances and those who are hemodynamically unstable. The use of nephrotoxic drugs should be limited as much as possible, and their necessity should be carefully assessed.

Miscellaneous Management Considerations

1. Red Blood Cell Transfusion: Transfusion is indicated when hemoglobin levels fall below 7.0 g/dL, unless specific conditions (e.g., myocardial infarction, severe hypoxaemia, acute hemorrhage) are present.

2. Glycaemic Control: If blood sugar levels exceed 10 mmol/L, glycaemic control is necessary. However, aiming for tighter blood sugar targets has been shown to increase the risk of hypoglycaemia without providing a mortality benefit. Management should focus on

avoiding both hypo- and hyperglycemia.

3. Procalcitonin: Procalcitonin levels can be useful in determining whether to discontinue antibiotics in patients with limited evidence of infection.

Post-Sepsis Syndrome (PSS)

Many patients who survive sepsis experience persistent symptoms such as muscle weakness, fatigue, joint pain, depression, anxiety, and difficulty concentrating or sleeping. These individuals may also have a weakened immune system, increasing their vulnerability to further infections. Up to one-third of sepsis survivors may require re-hospitalization within 3 months. Survivors should be closely monitored, with rehabilitation and support programs offered to help mitigate the effects of post-sepsis syndrome.

Chapter 6
Arterial blood gasses

Arterial blood gas (ABG) analysis is a critical diagnostic tool in emergency medicine, particularly for evaluating the respiratory and acid-base status of critically ill patients. Its accuracy and proper interpretation are essential for effective patient management.

Technical Aspects of Arterial Blood Gas Analysis

The development of arterial blood gas analysis began over 50 years ago with the creation of electrodes capable of measuring oxygen (PaO_2) and carbon dioxide ($PaCO_2$) partial pressures in arterial blood. The Clarke oxygen electrode is used to measure PaO_2 by detecting the current generated when oxygen molecules diffuse through a membrane and are reduced. Similarly, the Severinghaus CO_2 electrode measures $PaCO_2$ by assessing the change in pH as carbon dioxide interacts with water to produce hydrogen and bicarbonate ions.

The ABG analyzer calculates other important values such as bicarbonate concentration and base excess, which help assess acid-base balance. Modern blood gas analyzers also use co-oximetry to measure different forms of hemoglobin, including carboxyhemoglobin and methemoglobin, which can be important in diagnosing various conditions.

While blood gas analyzers usually report values at 37°C, adjustments for patient body temperature are often minimal and generally do not alter clinical decisions.

Collection and Handling of Blood Samples

Accurate ABG results depend on proper sample collection and handling. Blood samples should be collected in pretreated syringes to prevent coagulation and transported quickly to avoid changes in the sample's composition. Air bubbles or delayed processing can alter PaO_2, $PaCO_2$, and pH, as cellular metabolism continues in the sample, particularly in the presence of leucocytosis or thrombocytosis. Immediate cooling of the sample on ice can help stabilize it.

Arterial Puncture Technique

The radial artery is the most commonly used site for blood

collection due to its accessibility and the tolerability of the procedure. Other potential sites include the femoral, brachial, dorsalis pedis, and axillary arteries. The Modified Allen test is often used before radial artery puncture to ensure adequate collateral circulation from the ulnar artery, which is important to prevent ischemic complications.

Indwelling Arterial Catheters

In some cases, continuous blood pressure monitoring or frequent ABG sampling may require an indwelling arterial catheter. Proper aseptic techniques are essential during insertion and maintenance to prevent infections and other complications like bleeding, pseudoaneurysm formation, or ischemic injury due to thrombosis or embolism.

Interpretation of ABG Results

ABG analysis is integral in assessing gas exchange, ventilatory function, and acid-base balance in critically ill patients. The analysis provides insights into respiratory failure, whether related to oxygenation (hypoxemia) or ventilation (hypercapnia).

Gas Exchange and Respiratory Failure:

Effective gas exchange depends on the ability to deliver oxygen and remove carbon dioxide. Hypoxemia occurs when oxygen delivery is compromised, typically reflected in a PaO2 lower than 60 mm Hg. Hypercapnia results from impaired ventilation and can lead to respiratory acidosis. These issues often coexist in respiratory failure, which can be categorized into two types: Type I (hypoxemic) and Type II (hypercapnic). Type II is generally associated with inadequate alveolar ventilation due to factors such as poor respiratory drive, neuromuscular diseases, or lung/chest wall mechanical issues.

Alveolar–Arterial Oxygen Gradient:

The A–a gradient is calculated by determining the difference between the oxygen levels in the alveoli (PAO2) and arterial blood (PaO2). A higher A–a gradient indicates ventilation-perfusion mismatches, which are commonly seen in conditions like pneumonia or pulmonary embolism. The normal gradient is 5 to 15 mm Hg and can increase with smoking, age, or when higher levels of inspired oxygen are used.

Oxygen Delivery and Hemoglobin Saturation:

Oxygen delivery to tissues depends on the oxygen content in the blood, which is determined by hemoglobin saturation and the partial pressure of oxygen (PaO2). The oxygen content equation takes into account both the hemoglobin-bound oxygen and the dissolved oxygen in plasma. However, oxygen saturation (SaO2) is generally more important for assessing oxygen delivery than PaO2.

Oxygen-Hemoglobin Dissociation Curve:

The position of the oxygen-hemoglobin dissociation curve is influenced by factors such as PaCO2, pH, and body temperature. A rightward shift in the curve enhances oxygen delivery to tissues, which is beneficial during hypoxia. The P50 value, the PaO2 at which hemoglobin is 50% saturated with oxygen, is a useful reference.

Pathophysiology of Hypoxemic Respiratory Failure

Hypoxemic respiratory failure can be caused by several mechanisms, including impaired oxygen diffusion, shunting of blood, ventilation-perfusion mismatches, hypoventilation, and reduced oxygen availability. Identifying the underlying cause is essential for determining the most effective treatment.

Neurological Complications and Treatment Approaches Post-Cardiac Arrest

1. High Incidence of Neurological Injury: Neurological impairment following out-of-hospital cardiac arrest is frequent and is linked to considerable morbidity and mortality rates.

2. Impact of Reperfusion Injury: The successful

restoration of circulation after cardiac arrest results in the reperfusion of an ischemic brain. This triggers biochemical processes, largely driven by calcium influx, that lead to cellular damage and eventual cell death.

3. Uncertainty in Optimal Physiological Targets: The ideal targets for managing oxygenation, carbon dioxide levels, blood pressure, and temperature in the early stages after cardiac arrest remain uncertain. Current guidelines recommend maintaining these parameters within standard physiological ranges.

4. Lack of Effective Pharmacological Treatments: Presently, no specific medications have proven effective in enhancing neurological outcomes post-resuscitation.

Out-of-hospital cardiac arrest is a significant cause of mortality in developed nations. Prolonged arrest can induce global cerebral ischemia, leading to neurological injury. Many patients who achieve return of spontaneous circulation (ROSC) are comatose on arrival at the emergency department (ED) and subsequently require admission to the intensive care unit (ICU). A large proportion of these patients ultimately succumb to severe anoxic brain injury. Current global guidelines emphasize maintaining optimal levels of oxygenation, ventilation, blood pressure, and implementing targeted temperature management (TTM) to support these patients. This section delves into the mechanisms underlying neurological injury and explores emerging evidence on treatment strategies aimed at mitigating this injury and improving outcomes after cardiac arrest.

Pathophysiology of Cerebral Ischemia and Reperfusion Injury

The brain's high metabolic demand makes it acutely sensitive to decreases in oxygen and glucose supply. A reduction in cerebral oxygen delivery below 20 mL/100 g of brain tissue per minute shifts cellular metabolism to anaerobic pathways, significantly reducing adenosine triphosphate (ATP) production. Extended ischemia depletes ATP reserves, halting cellular metabolism, which disrupts the sodium-potassium pump and results in cellular swelling. This also causes metabolic acidosis due to hydrogen ion accumulation, which is detrimental to intracellular enzyme function.

Post-ROSC, reperfusion with oxygenated blood may cause additional harm. Increased intracellular glutamate levels, an excitatory neurotransmitter, activate calcium ion channels, causing calcium influx into cells. This triggers a cascade of biochemical reactions that generate free radicals and activate destructive enzymes, furthering cellular injury. Some neurons also undergo apoptosis, or programmed cell death, after the ischemic event. This delayed neuronal death varies by region, occurring within six hours in the striatum and up to seven days in hippocampal neurons, and is marked by cellular shrinkage, chromatin condensation, and DNA fragmentation.

Cerebral Hemodynamics Post-Reperfusion

Cerebral blood flow can remain impaired for hours following ROSC. Animal studies indicate an initial phase of hyperemia followed by decreased cerebral perfusion, even when systemic blood pressure is normalized. This is likely exacerbated by the inflammatory response, with factors like hypoxia, hypotension, and increased intracranial pressure contributing to reduced cerebral oxygenation. Increased metabolic demand due to fever or seizures can further compound this mismatch between oxygen supply and demand.

Exploration of Pharmacological Interventions

Several drugs that initially showed potential in reducing reperfusion injury in animal models have been tested in clinical trials, including thiopentone, corticosteroids, lidoflazine, nimodipine, magnesium, diazepam, and xenon gas. However, none of these interventions have demonstrated a clear improvement in neurological or overall survival outcomes over standard care. Clinical trials are ongoing to determine optimal oxygen, carbon dioxide, and temperature targets.

Oxygenation Strategy Post-Resuscitation

For patients who have undergone successful resuscitation after an out-of-hospital cardiac arrest but remain unconscious, paramedics administer 100% oxygen during transport to the ED. This approach, termed "hyperoxia," generally continues through ED admission, transfer, and into the ICU. After ICU admission, oxygen is gradually titrated to maintain a normal partial pressure of oxygen (pO2) between 70 and 100 mm Hg.

Animal studies, as well as large-scale observational studies, suggest that prolonged hyperoxia during the initial hours post-resuscitation may exacerbate neurological injury compared to lower oxygen levels. A study by Balan et al. demonstrated that animals exposed to controlled normoxia, with FiO2 titrated to achieve near-normal oxygen levels after ROSC, had improved neurological outcomes and reduced neuronal injury.

Clinical Evidence in Adults

Observational studies in adults support these findings, linking hyperoxia in ICU settings post-cardiac arrest with higher in-hospital mortality. In a study across 120 U.S. ICUs, patients with PaO2 levels above 300 mm Hg (hyperoxia) had significantly higher mortality rates compared to those with PaO2 levels in the normal range. Although adjustments were made for patient demographics and pre-existing conditions, hyperoxia remained associated with a higher risk of mortality.

Subsequent studies in Australian ICUs, both in- and

out-of-hospital cardiac arrest cases, revealed a similar association between hyperoxia and increased mortality. However, differences in oxygen administration protocols and data collection methods across studies indicate a need for further research to confirm these associations and establish optimal oxygenation strategies.

Neonatal Resuscitation and Oxygen Use

Evidence in neonatology has shown that resuscitating newborns with room air instead of 100% oxygen improves survival rates, leading to the adoption of room air as the standard in neonatal resuscitation.

Impact of Hyperoxia on Myocardial Injury

The AVOID trial highlighted the potential for increased myocardial injury with liberal oxygen administration in ST-elevation myocardial infarction (STEMI) patients. Among 441 patients, supplemental oxygen was linked to elevated creatine kinase and troponin levels, indicating greater myocardial damage. Given the prevalence of STEMI in comatose post-arrest patients, this evidence underscores the importance of cautious oxygen administration to limit potential myocardial and neurological damage during reperfusion.

Chapter 7
Anaphylaxis

Anaphylaxis is a severe and life-threatening hypersensitivity reaction that represents one of the most critical medical emergencies. It typically occurs abruptly in otherwise healthy individuals upon exposure to a specific trigger. Anaphylaxis can present along a spectrum, from mild symptoms to rapid and intense reactions that may involve multiple organ systems or manifest as isolated shock or respiratory distress. Immediate recognition and intervention with epinephrine, oxygen, and fluids are essential to stabilize the patient's cardiovascular and respiratory systems and improve outcomes. Appropriate discharge planning, including potential referral to an allergy specialist, is crucial in minimizing future anaphylactic episodes.

Definition

The term "anaphylaxis," coined by Richet and Portier in 1902, literally translates to "against protection" and refers to rapid, systemic, immunologically-driven responses that typically occur in previously sensitized individuals upon re-exposure to specific allergens. This type, known as immune-mediated or allergic anaphylaxis, contrasts with non-allergic anaphylaxis. Non-allergic anaphylaxis involves the release of similar inflammatory mediators but follows non-immunologic mechanisms and does not require prior sensitization. The World Allergy Organization (WAO) endorses the term "non-allergic anaphylaxis" over the older term "anaphylactoid reaction" to describe these cases. In this context, "anaphylaxis" will refer to both types of reactions, acknowledging their differing origins.

Classification of Anaphylaxis

The classification, diagnosis, and severity grading of anaphylaxis lack consistent international standards. Anaphylaxis is broadly defined as a serious, life-threatening, systemic hypersensitivity reaction. Both the National Institute of Allergy and Infectious Disease (NIAID) and the Food Allergy and Anaphylaxis Network (FAAN) define it as "a serious allergic reaction that is rapid in onset and may be fatal." NIAID and FAAN's detailed criteria encompass over 95% of clinical cases, dividing anaphylaxis diagnosis into three criteria to capture diverse presentations, including those without typical skin symptoms or with acute hypotensive episodes. Researchers are encouraged to use these comprehensive definitions while awaiting more refined diagnostic criteria from future prospective studies.

Severity Grading

Currently, there is no universally accepted grading system that aligns the clinical features of anaphylaxis with its severity, urgency, or treatment implications. However, a retrospective analysis of over 1,000 hypersensitivity reactions classified anaphylaxis into three grades. Mild reactions are often limited to skin and subcutaneous tissues, while moderate and severe reactions involve multiple systems and typically necessitate epinephrine, meeting the NIAID/FAAN criteria for anaphylaxis. This grading system offers a starting framework for descriptive research until more robust prospective data are available.

Etiology

Anaphylaxis commonly results from specific clinical triggers, including medications, biologics, insect stings, foods, anesthesia, natural rubber latex (NRL), exercise, and idiopathic cases. Certain risk factors—like comorbidities such as asthma, infection, physical exertion, alcohol intake, stress, or medications such as beta-blockers and ACE inhibitors—can increase susceptibility to anaphylaxis, referred to as "summation anaphylaxis."

ESSENTIAL POINTS

1. Anaphylaxis encompasses both immune-mediated (IgE-driven) and non-allergic, non-immunologic reactions. Comorbidities, concurrent medications, and triggers like asthma or stress heighten the risk.

2. Anaphylactic fatalities typically occur due to hypoxia from airway obstruction or bronchospasm, or from shock induced by vascular dilation and fluid shifts.

3. Parenteral penicillin, Hymenoptera stings, and certain foods are common triggers for IgE-mediated fatalities. Non-steroidal anti-inflammatory drugs (NSAIDs) and radiocontrast agents are primary culprits in non-allergic fatalities.

4. Epinephrine, oxygen, and fluid replacement are first-line treatments in anaphylaxis management.

5. H1 and H2 antihistamines, steroids, glucagon, and salbutamol are secondary

interventions once cardiovascular stability has been established with primary agents.

6. Patients should undergo a monitored recovery period of 4-6 hours post-anaphylaxis. Discharge protocols should include an epinephrine auto injector, a comprehensive action plan, and allergist referral if needed. Patient education is fundamental for long-term management.

7. Recently developed practice guidelines, such as those by the Joint Task Force on Practice Parameters (2015) and the European Academy of Allergy and Clinical Immunology (2014), offer comprehensive frameworks for anaphylaxis management.

Geographical Variation and Etiology

Geographic variations influence anaphylaxis prevalence; for instance, sesame allergy is more prevalent in the Middle East, while chickpea and rice allergies are more common in Asia. The most frequently cited anaphylactic triggers include penicillin, NSAIDs, chemotherapy agents, and monoclonal antibodies. Reactions to drugs like cisplatin, carboplatin, and specific monoclonal antibodies (e.g., omalizumab, cetuximab) are becoming more prevalent. Notably, cetuximab reactions may be linked to anti-galactose-alpha-1,3-galactose (α-gal) antibodies, with reactions sometimes delayed for hours.

Drug-Induced Anaphylaxis

Penicillin is the leading cause of drug-induced anaphylaxis, with an allergic reaction rate of approximately 1:500 courses. True allergic cross-reactivity between penicillin and first-generation cephalosporins is relatively rare, occurring in about 1-2% of patients. Reactions to NSAIDs are usually drug-specific, with minimal cross-reactivity among structurally dissimilar NSAIDs.

Insect Sting Anaphylaxis

Anaphylaxis from Hymenoptera stings (bees, wasps, ants) is second only to drug-induced anaphylaxis, impacting about 3% of adults and less than 1% of children. Fatal outcomes are more common in adults, frequently resulting from shock. In addition to anaphylactic reactions, large local reactions and serum sickness-like responses may follow stings.

Food-Induced Anaphylaxis

Food allergies, especially prevalent among younger populations, most frequently arise from the "Big 8" allergens: peanuts, tree nuts, shellfish, fish, milk, wheat, soy, and eggs. Cross-reactivity between food allergens varies and can be unpredictable. While fatalities are rare and often associated with asthma, biphasic reactions are possible, underscoring the importance of emergency preparedness and public education.

Perioperative and Latex-Induced Anaphylaxis

Anaphylaxis during anesthesia, frequently due to neuromuscular blocking agents, latex, antibiotics, and certain induction drugs, poses significant perioperative risks. High-risk groups for latex allergy include healthcare workers, children with congenital anomalies, and individuals with occupational exposure. Hospitals should have latex-free protocols to accommodate patients with known latex allergies.

Immune-Mediated Anaphylaxis (IgE and IgG4 Mechanisms)

Anaphylaxis primarily involves immune-mediated pathways, typically driven by IgE antibodies, and occasionally by IgG4. These antibodies are synthesized by plasma cells, originating from B lymphocytes under the regulation of helper T cells, following a prior sensitization to a specific antigen, though the precise mechanisms of this sensitization remain unclear. IgE antibodies attach to receptors on basophils and mast cells, effectively sensitizing them. Numerous agents can prompt IgE antibody production, including pharmaceuticals, biological agents, foods, insect venoms, and environmental allergens.

Non-IgE-Mediated Anaphylaxis

Non-IgE-mediated anaphylaxis occurs independently of IgE antibodies. Instead, various stimuli directly trigger mediator release, complement activation, or engage the clotting and fibrinolysis systems. Physical stimuli, medications, biological agents, and food additives can all precipitate these non-allergic responses.

Cellular Activation and Mediator Release

When allergens cross-link surface IgE Fc receptors (FcεRI) on sensitized basophils and mast cells, these cells release inflammatory mediators. This process is further fueled by an influx of calcium ions, which facilitates the release of pre-stored mediators and the synthesis of new lipid-based inflammatory molecules. Key mediators released include histamine, proteases, prostaglandins, leukotrienes, cytokines, and chemokines, which together contribute to the intense inflammatory response in anaphylaxis.

Modulation of Mediator Release

Mediator release within cells is regulated by intracellular cyclic AMP (cAMP) levels, with substances that increase cAMP, like epinephrine, inhibiting mediator release. This explains the central role of epinephrine in managing anaphylaxis, as it counteracts the effects of mediator release.

Pharmacological Effects of Mediators

Anaphylactic mediators drive vasodilation, enhance capillary permeability, and stimulate glandular secretion, leading to symptoms such as smooth muscle contraction, especially in the bronchi. Additionally, these mediators recruit further immune cells, including eosinophils and neutrophils, establishing a self-perpetuating inflammatory cascade.

Clinical Manifestations of Anaphylaxis

Cutaneous Symptoms

Anaphylaxis often presents with skin-related symptoms,

including a warm, tingling sensation, a sense of anxiety, generalized erythema, urticaria, pruritus, and angioedema. These early signs, noted in 80-90% of cases, are essential for prompt diagnosis but can sometimes be absent due to early intervention or subtle presentation.

Systemic and Respiratory Symptoms

Anaphylaxis is marked by rapid involvement of multiple organ systems, including the respiratory and cardiovascular systems. Respiratory symptoms such as throat tightness, coughing, and severe bronchospasm can lead to critical distress. Hypoxia, indicated by an oxygen saturation below 92%, is a hallmark of severe anaphylaxis requiring immediate intervention.

Cardiovascular and Neurological Manifestations

Systemic involvement may also include lightheadedness, sweating, syncope, or coma, often accompanied by tachycardia, hypotension, and arrhythmias. In some cases, coronary artery spasm can cause chest pain, even without preexisting coronary disease, due to the release of mediators from cardiac mast cells.

Gastrointestinal Symptoms

Gastrointestinal distress, including difficulty swallowing, nausea, vomiting, diarrhea, and cramps, can occur in up to one-third of cases, though these symptoms are typically secondary to more life-threatening complications.

Differential Diagnosis

The wide array of anaphylactic symptoms necessitates careful differentiation from other conditions. Asthma, pulmonary edema, foreign body inhalation, and irritant chemical exposure may present with similar respiratory symptoms. Vasovagal responses, other types of shock, scombroid poisoning, carcinoid syndrome, ACE inhibitor-induced angioedema, and hereditary C1 esterase inhibitor deficiency are all potential differential diagnoses that require thorough assessment.

Clinical Investigations and Laboratory Assessment

Anaphylaxis is clinically diagnosed, with laboratory testing reserved for ambiguous cases. Pulse oximetry, electrolyte assessment, and blood gas analysis are useful for tracking disease progression. Mast cell tryptase levels, ideally measured at specific intervals, can support diagnosis, though they are not definitive on their own.

Revised Analysis of Anaphylaxis Management

Antihistamine Use and Limitations

Antihistamines alone should not be the primary treatment for severe anaphylaxis. H1-antihistamines may cause adverse effects, such as sedation, confusion, and vasodilation, particularly when administered intravenously. Combining H1- and H2-antihistamines has shown to be more effective in reducing skin symptoms in allergic reactions than using an H1-antagonist by itself. For post-discharge use, a non-sedating H1-antihistamine (e.g., loratadine 10 mg daily) may be preferred, especially for patients who need to work or drive (refer to discharge guidelines).

Role of Corticosteroids

The efficacy of corticosteroids in acute anaphylaxis remains uncertain due to a lack of placebo-controlled studies. Despite theoretical benefits on inflammation and tissue reactivity, such as mitigating late-phase eosinophilic responses, corticosteroids are commonly used due to their safety profile. For patients with airway symptoms or bronchospasm, prednisone (1 mg/kg up to 50 mg orally) or hydrocortisone (1.5 -- 3 mg/kg IV) is typically administered, informed by corticosteroids' established role in asthma. Although steroids may help prevent biphasic reactions (symptom recurrence post-recovery), the supporting evidence is weak. However, corticosteroids are crucial for managing recurrent idiopathic anaphylaxis.

Glucagon, Atropine, and Salbutamol in β-blocked Patients

Patients on β-blockers may experience more severe or treatment-resistant anaphylaxis. If adrenaline fails, glucagon (1–5 mg IV followed by 5–15 μg/min titrated) can be administered, as it increases cyclic AMP through a non-adrenergic pathway. Side effects include nausea and vomiting. Some patients with anaphylactic shock may experience adrenaline-resistant bradycardia, potentially due to neurocardiogenic reflexes, where atropine (0.6 mg IV, up to 0.02 mg/kg) has shown efficacy. Salbutamol nebulization may be added to adrenaline to address bronchospasm, offering a familiar therapeutic option.

Alternative Vasopressors

For cases of hypotension unresponsive to adrenaline and fluid replacement, alternative vasopressors like noradrenaline, metaraminol, phenylephrine, or vasopressin may be beneficial.

Methylene Blue for Vasodilation

In nitric oxide-mediated vasodilation resistant to other therapies, methylene blue (1.5–2.0 mg/kg) may help, though rare cases of anaphylaxis due to methylene blue itself have been documented.

Pretreatment Recommendations

Routine prophylactic administration of corticosteroids or antihistamines to prevent severe reactions, such as with contrast media during imaging procedures, is generally unreliable and not recommended based on current literature.

Observation and Disposition

Patients treated for systemic anaphylactic reactions, including those receiving adrenaline, should be monitored for 4–6 hours post-recovery. Extended observation (8–10 hours) is advisable for individuals with prolonged reactions, oral allergen exposure, reactive airway disease, or heart conditions, as fatalities in these groups are higher. Observation can safely occur in the emergency department if appropriate facilities are available; ECG monitoring is not necessary. Patients with unstable vital signs or those responding poorly to adrenaline may require ICU admission.

Biphasic Anaphylaxis

Biphasic anaphylaxis, which occurs in 1–5% of cases, involves recurrence after initial symptom resolution. Factors potentially contributing to biphasic response include severe initial presentation, delays in adrenaline administration, inadequate doses, and lack of steroid use. Observation of 4–6 hours is typically sufficient, though higher-risk patients (e.g., asthmatics, oral allergen exposure, heart disease) may require 8–10 hours.

Discharge Protocol

Following observation, assess the need for take-home medications, a self-injectable adrenaline device, and possible referral to an allergist or immunologist. For patients with significant skin reactions or bronchospasm, consider loratadine 10 mg once daily, ranitidine 150 mg every 12 hours, and prednisolone 50 mg/day for a brief period (2–3 days).

Self-Injectable Adrenaline Devices

Self-injectable adrenaline is advised for patients at risk of future anaphylaxis, particularly those with food allergies (e.g., nuts), unknown anaphylaxis triggers, or reactions occurring outside of medical settings. The choice between EpiPen and Anapen (0.3 mg for adults, 0.15 mg for children) should be based on availability and the patient's familiarity with administration techniques. Each device's use should be clearly demonstrated to the patient and caregivers, and they should be informed about proper storage and shelf-life considerations (1–2 years).

Allergist/Immunologist Referral

An allergist or immunologist referral is recommended for patients prescribed self-injectable adrenaline, those with severe reactions, and cases of insect sting allergies potentially eligible for immunotherapy. Referral documentation should include reaction details and suspected triggers. Patients should also maintain a detailed record of foods, medications, and exposures preceding the reaction, as accurate recall diminishes over time.

Precautions for Recurrence

Patients susceptible to anaphylaxis should avoid β-blockers when possible, as well as ACE inhibitors in hypertensive or ischemic heart disease cases, after consulting with relevant specialists. Minimizing allergen exposure through preventive actions, such as removing wasp nests and carefully reading food labels, can also reduce risk.

Allergen Testing

Allergen testing, including IgE skin and in vitro tests, should be conducted only by experienced professionals to ensure accuracy and patient safety. Skin prick tests offer higher sensitivity and are preferred when using standardized extracts. Testing should be done 3–4 weeks post-episode, under allergist or immunologist supervision, given the potential for severe reactions.

References

1. Nolan JP, Hazinski MF, Aickin R, et al. Executive summary on the 2015 guidelines for cardiopulmonary resuscitation and emergency cardiovascular care. Resuscitation. 2015;95:e1–e31.

2. Cummins RO, Ornato JP, Thies WH, Pepe PE. Concept of the "Chain of Survival" for enhancing survival rates from sudden cardiac arrest. Circulation. 1991;83(5):1832–1847.

3. Travers AH, Perkins GD, Berg RA, et al. Adult BLS and AED guidelines from the 2015 International Consensus. Circulation. 2015;132(16 Suppl 1):S51–S83.

4. Beck B, Bray J, Cameron P, et al. Out-of-hospital cardiac arrest statistics in Australia and

New Zealand. Resuscitation. 2018;126:49–57.

5. Wang PL, Brooks SC. Comparative study of mechanical versus manual chest compressions in cardiac arrest. Cochrane Database of Systematic Reviews. 2018;8:Cd007260.

6. Flato UA, Paiva EF, Carballo MT, et al. Role of echocardiography in ICU patients with non-shockable rhythm cardiac arrest. Resuscitation. 2015;92:1–6.

7. Hagihara A, Hasegawa M, Abe T, et al. Prehospital epinephrine and its impact on cardiac arrest survival. JAMA. 2012;307(11):1161–1168.

8. Perkins GD, Ji C, Deakin CD, Quinn T, et al. Clinical trial on epinephrine's effects in out-of-hospital cardiac arrest cases. New England Journal of Medicine. 2018;379(8):711–721.

9. Chowdhury A, Fernandes B, Melhuish TM, White LD. Analysis of antiarrhythmic drugs in cardiac arrest. Heart Lung Circulation. 2018;27(3):280–290.

10. Khan SU, Winnicka L, Saleem MA, Rahman H, Rehman N. Bayesian meta-analysis on amiodarone, lidocaine, and magnesium in ventricular arrhythmias. Heart Lung. 2017;46(6):417–424.

11. Sasson C, Hegg AJ, Macy M, et al. Termination criteria for resuscitation in out-of-hospital cardiac arrests. JAMA. 2008;300(12):1432–1438.

12. Simons, F.E.R., Ardusso, L., Bilò, B. (2011). World Allergy Organization's assessment and management guidelines for anaphylaxis. Journal of Allergy and Clinical Immunology, 127, 593.

13. Galli, S.J. (2005). An overview of anaphylaxis pathogenesis and management challenges. Journal of Allergy and Clinical Immunology, 115, 571–574.

14. Sampson, H.A., Munoz-Furlong, A., Campbell, R.L., et al. (2006). Summary of the second NIAID/FAAN symposium on anaphylaxis definition and management. Journal of Allergy and Clinical Immunology, 117, 391–397.

15. Brown, S.G.A. (2004). Clinical features and a grading system for anaphylaxis severity. Journal of Allergy and Clinical Immunology, 114, 371–376.

16. Lieberman, P., Nicklas, R., Randolph, C., et al. (2015). Updated practice guidelines for anaphylaxis management. Annals of Allergy, Asthma & Immunology, 115, 341–384.

17. Sheikh, A., Ten Broek, V., Brown, S.G.A., et al. (2007). Use of H1-antihistamines in anaphylaxis treatment. Cochrane Database of Systematic Reviews, 1, CD006160.

18. Choo, K., Simons, F., Sheikh, A. (2012). The role of glucocorticoids in managing anaphylaxis. Cochrane Database of Systematic Reviews, 4, CD007596.

19. Vale, S., Smith, J., Loh, R. (2012). Recommendations for safe adrenaline autoinjector use. Australian Prescriber, 35, 56–58.

20. Pumphrey, R.S.H. (2000). Insights from fatal anaphylaxis cases to improve management

practices. Clinical and Experimental Allergy, 30, 1144–1150.

Chapter 8 (A)
Trauma

Epidemiology of Trauma

Trauma accounts for approximately 9% of all global deaths, with motor vehicle accidents ranking as a leading cause of both death and disability-adjusted life years (DALYs) lost. Notably, in high-income nations, trauma is the primary cause of mortality for individuals aged 1–44. This burden is even more pronounced in developing countries where trauma care infrastructure is often underdeveloped or non-existent. Unintentional injuries, such as those from road accidents, typically result in more fatalities than intentional injuries like suicide or homicide. However, in some regions, such as Australia, suicide has surpassed motor vehicle accidents as a leading cause of death in certain age groups (15–44 years). The economic and social ramifications of trauma are substantial, particularly as it frequently affects young individuals who play active roles in society.

Advances in Trauma Systems

In many developed nations, a systematic approach to trauma care has led to marked reductions in injury-related mortality and morbidity. Prevention initiatives—such as seatbelt mandates, drink-driving laws, improved road infrastructure, helmet requirements for motorcyclists and bicyclists, and public awareness campaigns on road and workplace safety—have contributed significantly to these improvements. Additionally, changes in trauma care systems and patient management have further enhanced survival rates, although prevention remains the most effective measure.

The initial exploration of trauma care in the United States was driven by the high prevalence of urban violence and road trauma, alongside insights gained from military conflicts in the 20th century. Researchers, including Trunkey, categorized trauma deaths into a trimodal distribution. Approximately 50% of fatalities occur within the first hour due to severe vascular or neurological injuries, underscoring the need for prevention. Another 30% of deaths occur later, primarily from respiratory and circulatory issues caused by major truncal injuries. The final 20% happen in the days following the injury due to complications such as acute respiratory distress syndrome (ARDS), multiple organ failure (MOF), sepsis, and brain injury. Trauma system advancements have successfully reduced the percentage of fatalities within the second category through timely and organized intervention.

Key Elements of a Trauma Care System

1. Primary Objectives: The primary goal of a well-functioning trauma system is rapid identification and transfer of severely injured patients to

appropriate care facilities in minimal time.

2. Initial Patient Management: Trauma management begins with a team-based approach and a structured primary survey, addressing critical aspects like airway, breathing, circulation, disability, and exposure (ABCDE). This is followed by a comprehensive secondary examination.

3. Continuous Quality Improvement: Regular audits and performance feedback within trauma systems are essential for achieving optimal patient outcomes.

The Trauma System: Pre-Hospital and In-Hospital Phases

Pre-Hospital Care: While initial trauma care research prioritized specialized centers, the importance of pre-hospital care is now recognized as central to trauma outcomes. In mature trauma systems, timely prehospital interventions and proper triage to facilities capable of managing severe injuries are critical. High-risk patients benefit from transport to specialized hospitals with advanced trauma care capabilities. Pre-hospital teams, which may include paramedics or physicians, are often trained to perform advanced procedures like intubation and chest decompression to stabilize patients before arrival at the hospital.

In-Hospital Trauma Response: Effective pre-hospital communication enables hospitals to prepare for trauma patient arrivals, facilitating the organization of trauma teams and setup of trauma bays. Upon arrival, trauma teams employ systematic assessment protocols (such as those taught in Advanced Trauma Life Support, or ATLS) to manage life-threatening injuries.

Essential Management Phases in Trauma Care

1. Airway Management: Given the high risk of hypoxia in trauma patients, early airway intervention by skilled personnel is essential. Methods such as suction, removal of foreign bodies, or jaw-thrust maneuvers are employed to

maintain a patent airway. Endotracheal intubation is recommended for patients at risk of airway compromise.

2. Breathing: Post-airway stabilization, ensuring adequate ventilation and oxygenation is prioritized. Immediate attention is directed toward addressing any life-threatening respiratory issues, including pneumothorax or flail chest, to optimize breathing and gas exchange.

Shock, a serious clinical condition, arises when vital organs do not receive adequate blood flow to sustain function. In trauma patients, severe blood loss is often the main culprit. However, other less frequent causes of shock should also be considered, including:

Tension Pneumothorax: Rapidly compromises circulation.

Cardiogenic Shock: May result from pre-existing conditions (e.g., acute myocardial infarction leading to trauma, medications causing reduced cardiac compensation, or hypovolemia) or from direct cardiac injury, such as myocardial contusion, valve/septal damage, or pericardial tamponade.

Neurogenic Shock: Caused by loss of sympathetic tone, it may stem from brain stem injuries, spinal cord trauma, or vasomotor instability. Bradycardia is a hallmark but may also occur in severe hypovolemia.

Anaphylactic and Septic Shock: These may coincide with hypovolemic shock, compounding the condition.

Identifying the initial stages of hypovolemic shock can be challenging. Relying solely on systolic blood pressure is insufficient, and all patients at risk of substantial blood loss, even with a seemingly minor possibility, should be closely monitored. Early assessment of clinical parameters offers insights into organ perfusion, but more invasive monitoring may be essential in severe cases.

Immediate action is required if there is significant visible hemorrhage, involving measures such as applying direct pressure, wound closure, or using a tourniquet. Rapid venous access is crucial, typically achieved with two large-bore peripheral lines; central venous access may be necessary if arm veins are not accessible. Optimal site selection depends on several factors: the subclavian vein is reliable for patency, femoral access can be effective but has limitations in cases of major trunk bleeding, and the internal jugular vein is challenging in immobilized patients. Alternative approaches include using the saphenous veins or cubital fossa.

Initially, crystalloids are generally sufficient for managing suspected blood loss when blood pressure is stable. Evidence does not favor non-blood colloids vs crystalloids, nor does it clearly support hypertonic crystalloids. However, if hypotension and tachycardia are present, immediate blood transfusion is required, starting with O-negative blood and transitioning to matched blood when available. Over-resuscitation should be avoided until bleeding is controlled, as excessive fluid resuscitation may worsen outcomes. Tranexamic acid (TXA) may also benefit patients with hemorrhagic shock.

After securing the airway and ensuring oxygenation, achieving definitive hemorrhage control is the key to survival in major trauma patients. Delaying surgery to restore normal intravascular volume is unnecessary. Identifying the bleeding source—commonly the chest, abdomen, pelvis, long bones, or scalp—is a priority.

Disability

During the primary assessment, identifying potential head injuries is critical. Consciousness levels are evaluated using the Glasgow Coma Scale, alongside neurological signs (pupil response, limb weakness). Suspected intracranial injuries warrant immediate CT imaging upon completion of the initial evaluation.

Exposure and Temperature Control

Hypothermia can lead to worse outcomes in trauma patients, so maintaining normal body temperature is essential to avoid metabolic imbalances and coagulation issues. However, using therapeutic hypothermia in head injuries remains debated. Full exposure, including log-rolling with spinal immobilization, allows for thorough examination without risking hypothermia.

Next Steps and Specialized Care

Following initial life-saving measures, a cohesive and skilled trauma team continues the assessment. Additional specialists, such as orthopedic surgeons or neurosurgeons, may be needed depending on the evolving clinical picture. Immediate imaging should include targeted x-rays, such as AP chest and pelvis views, ideally within the resuscitation area to avoid moving an unstable patient. Ultrasound is increasingly valuable for detecting life-threatening conditions like internal bleeding or cardiac tamponade. After the primary survey and necessary imaging, a secondary survey involves a complete history and a head-to-toe examination to identify any less obvious injuries. Coordinated care is essential, with a team leader overseeing the patient's treatment throughout the hospital stay. Effective handover to the ongoing care provider is vital for continuous, high-quality trauma management.

Quality Improvement in Trauma Care

Trauma outcomes vary, but examining trauma deaths from a public health perspective reveals preventable causes. Trauma Quality Improvement (TQI) programs aim to identify care gaps, implement corrective actions like protocols and targeted training, and track improvements through tools like trauma registries. These registries collect data on injury severity, physiological response, and patient demographics, allowing meaningful outcome comparisons.

Trauma in Developing Countries

Developing countries increasingly recognize the substantial human and economic toll of trauma, especially from road accidents. Public health initiatives, such as seatbelt and helmet regulations, mirror strategies in developed countries. Evidence shows that trauma system implementation significantly reduces preventable deaths. Trauma registries are crucial for assessing outcomes and tracking the impact of system improvements. Additionally, standardized trauma education programs, like ATLS and Primary Trauma Care (PTC), play a vital role in providing essential skills in resource-limited settings.

Neurotrauma

Neurotrauma is a prevalent condition in cases of multisystem trauma, particularly in incidents such as motor vehicle accidents and falls. Head injuries account for

30% to 50% of all trauma-related fatalities. This presents a significant burden on healthcare systems, with hospital admissions for head trauma reaching up to 300 per 100,000 people annually, and this figure doubles among the elderly. The long-term effects of moderate to severe neurotrauma significantly drain healthcare resources, and even mild brain injuries now show clearer links to prolonged morbidity. Despite advancements in preventive strategies, trauma systems, resuscitative therapies, and rehabilitation, neurotrauma remains a critical health concern due to the long-term disability it causes, affecting the quality of life and societal productivity.

Pathogenesis

Primary brain injury results directly from the mechanical forces of the traumatic incident and can be mitigated through preventive measures like helmet use. Secondary brain injury, which occurs within 2 to 24 hours of the initial trauma, involves a complex series of biological responses. A major mechanism is cerebral hypoxia, caused by impaired oxygenation or cerebral blood flow. Cerebral perfusion pressure (CPP), mean arterial pressure (MAP), and intracranial pressure (ICP) regulate blood flow to the brain, with raised ICP from hemorrhage or cerebral edema further compromising blood flow. Other factors, such as cerebral vasospasm from significant subarachnoid hemorrhage, exacerbate the injury.

Cellular dysfunction from both primary and secondary injury involves disturbances in ion balances (sodium, calcium, magnesium, potassium), the generation of oxygen free radicals, lipid peroxidation, and excitotoxicity due to excessive neurotransmitter release, especially glutamate. These factors contribute to brain cell damage and function loss.

Classification of Primary Neurotrauma Injuries

Primary injuries can be classified into several categories:

Skull Fractures: The significance lies not just in the bone injury but in the associated neurotrauma. For instance, fractures near the middle meningeal artery are linked to extradural hemorrhage, while skull base fractures may lead to cerebrospinal fluid (CSF) leaks and infection risks. Depressed skull fractures can compress underlying structures, causing secondary brain injury that might require surgical intervention.

Concussion: This is a temporary alteration in brain function, often marked by a loss of consciousness (LOC). While recovery is typically rapid, post-concussion symptoms, such as headaches and mild cognitive disturbances, may persist. "Second-impact syndrome" can occur, where a second injury after a concussion leads to severe cerebral swelling, which is dangerous. Some animal models suggest that concussion can also result in temporary increases in ICP and cell function disturbances.

Contusion: A brain bruise that occurs when forces lower than those required for shearing injuries cause tissue damage. The size and location of the contusion, especially in the frontal or temporal lobes, dictate the morbidity. Larger contusions can lead to hematomas, edema, or seizures.

Intracranial Hematomas: These can be classified into several types:

Extradural Hematoma (EDH): Often caused by temporal bone fractures damaging the middle meningeal artery, EDH can lead to raised ICP and herniation if untreated.

Subdural Hematoma (SDH): This typically results from moderate trauma, especially in elderly individuals or children. It can present as acute, subacute, or chronic, with the latter having a lower mortality.

Intracerebral Hemorrhage (ICH): Blood vessels within the brain rupture, typically in the temporal or posterior frontal lobes, leading to varying functional impairments depending on the hemorrhage location.

Subarachnoid and Intraventricular Hemorrhages: These are relatively common in severe trauma and may lead to cerebral vasospasm and secondary ischemic injury.

Diffuse Axonal Injury (DAI): DAI is caused by rotational and shearing forces that damage axonal connections within the brain. It occurs in up to 50% of neurotrauma cases and can cause long-term neurological deficits even when CT scans appear normal. The mechanism involves microscopic disruptions in communication pathways, particularly in the corpus callosum and midbrain.

Penetrating Injury: High-morbidity injuries, such as gunshot wounds, expose cerebral tissue and are associated with poor prognosis, especially when the injury involves the skull base or the periorbital/perinasal regions.

Epidemiology

Neurotrauma is a leading cause of death and disability, with traumatic brain injury (TBI) affecting more than 30% of the population in certain settings. Approximately 40% of individuals with TBI will have lasting disabilities. Common causes of TBI include motor vehicle accidents, falls, assaults, and firearms, with alcohol often being a factor in young male cases.

Prevention

Preventing neurotrauma involves both primary and secondary strategies. Primary prevention focuses on reducing the causes of trauma, such as implementing speed limits, promoting vehicle safety measures, and encouraging the use of helmets. Secondary prevention seeks to limit the damage after the injury, primarily through maintaining adequate cerebral perfusion and oxygenation, as detailed in the clinical management section.

Clinical Features

Definition and Classification of TBI

For decades, TBI has been classified into mild, moderate, or severe categories based on the Glasgow Coma Scale (GCS). Recent advancements have led to additional systems that more accurately define TBI severity, especially for mild cases. The contemporary classifications include:

Definite Moderate-Severe TBI: Defined by death, a GCS score below 13, LOC greater than 30 minutes, post-traumatic amnesia (PTA) longer than 24 hours, or imaging evidence of brain injury.

Probable Mild TBI: GCS > 12, LOC < 30 minutes, PTA < 24 hours.

Possible Mild TBI: Symptoms like confusion, dizziness, or nausea without a clear history of LOC.

History and Primary Survey

A thorough history of the trauma's mechanics is essential for managing moderate to severe TBI. This history helps in understanding the injury's progression, associated comorbidities, and pre-existing health issues. In trauma care, the initial focus should be on maintaining airway, ventilation, and adequate circulatory pressure (CPP) according to Advanced Trauma Life Support (ATLS) protocols. The most significant risks for patients with severe head injuries are hypoxia and inadequate cerebral perfusion.

Indications for Intubation and Ventilation

Ventilation support is required if a patient experiences inadequate gas exchange (hypercarbia, hypoxia), difficulty maintaining airway integrity, or when transport is necessary, and the airway may be unstable. Elevated ICP requires elevated systemic blood pressure to support cerebral perfusion. Hypotensive resuscitation strategies are not suitable for neurotrauma patients. Early neurological assessment using the GCS or AVPU scale is critical for monitoring neurological status. Hypoxia ($PaO_2 < 60$ mmHg or 8 kPa) should be promptly addressed to prevent further complications. The management of intracranial pressure (ICP) plays a critical role in the acute treatment of neurotrauma, with the primary aim being the prevention of secondary brain injury and associated cerebral swelling.

ICP monitoring is typically recommended for patients with severe head injury (Glasgow Coma Scale [GCS] < 9) who remain unconscious. There are variations in institutional practices regarding the methods of ICP measurement and the specific indications for monitoring. In certain cases, the use of cerebrospinal fluid (CSF) drainage to reduce ICP may be considered for patients with an initial GCS of less than 6 within the first 12 hours post-injury. Elevating the head of the bed to 30 degrees has been shown to modestly reduce ICP without significantly affecting cerebral perfusion pressure (CPP).

Mannitol (0.25–1.0 g/kg IV) may offer temporary relief by reducing ICP, although there is no substantial evidence supporting its impact on long-term patient outcomes. This osmotic agent can lead to non-selective osmotic dehydration and may cause complications such as fluid overload, hyperosmolality, hypovolemia, and rebound cerebral edema. It can be used as a short-term measure to stabilize patients before surgery.

Routine hyperventilation in cases of head injury is discouraged, as hypocarbia can decrease cerebral blood flow (and ICP) through vasoconstriction. This effect, if excessive, can reduce CPP to levels that exacerbate secondary brain injury.

Anticonvulsant prophylaxis with phenytoin (loading dose of 15–18 mg/kg IV over 30–60 minutes) is recommended to prevent seizures in the first week post-injury. Although levetiracetam is being explored, there is insufficient evidence to recommend it over phenytoin. Acute seizures are managed according to standard guidelines, including the use of benzodiazepines. Intubation and mechanical ventilation may be necessary for status epilepticus or refractory seizures.

Antibiotic prophylaxis is indicated for compound fractures, and tetanus immunization is part of standard wound care. While ongoing research is investigating cerebral protective therapies, there is currently no evidence supporting the use of steroids in head injury management, and they are not recommended. Bifrontal decompressive craniectomy, though not shown to improve long-term outcomes in severe diffuse traumatic brain injury (TBI), can effectively reduce ICP and shorten ICU stay.

The use of hypothermia remains controversial. While animal studies suggest potential benefits, human trials have shown mixed or inconclusive results, and prophylactic hypothermia is not currently recommended. High-dose barbiturates may be employed to manage refractory elevated

ICP when conventional medical and surgical treatments fail.

In summary, general supportive care—maintaining thermoregulation, hydration, pressure care, and nutrition—remains the cornerstone of neurotrauma management.

Disposition

For patients with mild TBI, recommendations regarding the appropriate observation period, the need for hospitalization, and the predictive value of injury mechanisms are inconsistent. Managing these cases in rural or isolated settings can present logistical challenges. In such cases, extended observation, combined with early neurosurgical consultation and a low threshold for transfer to a specialized center, is advisable.

Patients with moderate to severe neurotrauma should be admitted to the hospital, ideally under the care of a neurosurgeon in a specialized neurocritical care unit. Early rehabilitation and social reintegration should be integrated into the treatment plan.

Transfer of patients with significant neurotrauma to other hospitals must be performed by skilled personnel, ensuring continuity of care. Airway management during transfer must anticipate potential deterioration. The presence of pneumocephalus contraindicates unpressurized high-altitude flight. Teleradiology and remote neurosurgical consultation can significantly aid in managing patients with head injuries in isolated locations.

References

1. Muraro, A., Roberts, G., Worm, M. (2014). European Academy of Allergy and Clinical Immunology's guidelines on anaphylaxis management. Allergy, 69, 1026–1045.

2. Kaukonen, K., Bailey, M., Suzuki, S., et al. (2014). Analysis of mortality associated with severe sepsis and septic shock in critically ill patients in Australia and New Zealand from 2000 to 2012. JAMA, 311(13), 1308.

3. Singer, M., Deutschman, C., Seymour, C., et al. (2016). The Sepsis-3 consensus definitions for sepsis and septic shock. JAMA, 315(8), 801–810.

4. ProCESS Investigators, Yealy, D.M., Kellum, J.A., et al. (2014). Evaluation of protocol-based interventions in early septic shock management through a randomized trial. New England Journal of Medicine, 370(18), 1683–1693.

5. ARISE Investigators; ANZICS Clinical Trials Group, Peake, S.L., et al. (2014). Study on goal-directed resuscitation in early septic shock patients. New England Journal of Medicine, 371(16), 1496–1506.

6. Mouncey, P., Osborn, T., Power, G., et al. (2015). A trial comparing early, goal-directed resuscitation strategies for septic shock treatment. New England Journal of Medicine, 372(14), 1301–1311.

7. Venkatesh, B., Finfer, S., Cohen, J., et al. (2018). Evaluating the impact of adjunctive glucocorticoid therapy in septic shock patients.

New England Journal of Medicine, 378(9), 797–808.

8. Annane, D., Renault, A., Brun-Buisson, C., et al. (2018). Efficacy of combined hydrocortisone and fludrocortisone therapy in adults with septic shock. New England Journal of Medicine, 378(9), 809–818.

9. Griesdale, D., de Souza, R., van Dam, R., et al. (2009). Meta-analysis on intensive insulin therapy and mortality in critically ill patients, incorporating NICE-SUGAR study data. Canadian Medical Association Journal, 180(8), 821–827.

10. Prescott, H., Angus, D. (2018). Examining long-term morbidity following sepsis. JAMA, 319(1), 91.

11. Serafim, R., Gomes, J., Salluh, J., Póvoa, P. (2018). Comparative study of quick-SOFA and SIRS criteria for sepsis diagnosis and mortality prediction. Chest, 153(3), 646–655.

Chapter 8 (B)
Spinal trauma

ESSENTIALS

1. In conscious, alert patients under 65, clinically significant cervical spine injuries can generally be ruled out using clinical examination criteria alone, as outlined in the National Emergency X-Radiography Utilization Study (NEXUS) and the Canadian C-spine rules.

2. Physical examination alone is not sufficient for diagnosing unstable vertebral injuries, unless there is a gross deformity.

3. The absence of neurological symptoms does not rule out spinal column injuries or the potential for spinal cord damage.

4. A patient may be able to walk and still have a serious vertebral injury, including one that could be unstable.

5. The progression of spinal cord injury may result in worsening symptoms, which may not appear until hours after the initial trauma.

6. Magnetic resonance imaging (MRI) is becoming the preferred imaging technique for patients presenting with

neurological symptoms, due to its ability to provide detailed images of the spinal cord.

7. In unconscious trauma victims, the probability of significant vertebral injury is about 10%, with 2% of all patients with altered consciousness suffering from spinal cord injury.

8. Although spinal immobilization is a key part of care to prevent further injury, it can lead to complications if not used properly.

9. Methylprednisolone is generally not recommended for use in most Australian and international centers for spinal cord injuries; however, if administered, it should be within 8 hours of the injury to potentially improve motor function and overall outcomes.

Introduction

Spinal cord injury (SCI) is a devastating trauma, often resulting in permanent physical and psychological impairments. It disrupts not only the individual's life but also impacts their family, friends, and broader community.

Around 2% of adults experiencing blunt trauma suffer from SCI, with the risk increasing threefold in patients with craniofacial injuries. The primary causes of acute SCI in Australia include motor vehicle accidents, falls, and certain sports injuries, particularly diving and water activities. Road traffic accidents alone account for nearly half of spinal injuries, while despite efforts to reduce risks in contact sports like rugby, significant injuries continue to occur. Younger individuals are particularly vulnerable, but even minor falls in older adults or low-impact trauma in those with pre-existing bone conditions can lead to SCI. Notably, pathological vertebral fractures may sometimes be the first sign of malignancy.

Two studies have highlighted the potential for preventable neurological deterioration due to factors such as:

Failure to recognize the injury initially, either due to inadequate examination or other injuries masking the SCI

Secondary injury effects such as oedema or ischaemia

Further damage to the spinal cord from insufficient oxygenation or hypotension

Aggravation of the injury from improper immobilization of the vertebral column

Pathophysiology

Level of Vertebral Injury

Studies from Victoria and New South Wales show that spinal injuries predominantly occur in the cervical (60%), thoracic (30%), lumbar (4%), and sacral (2%) regions. The cervical spine, particularly the 5th, 6th, and 7th vertebrae, is more susceptible to injury due to its greater mobility. The C5-C6 and C6-C7 levels are responsible for nearly half of all cervical subluxations resulting from blunt trauma.

Associated Injuries

Observations reveal several key findings in patients with SCI:

1. About 8% to 10% of those with a vertebral fracture will sustain a second fracture, often at a distant site. These secondary injuries are typically minor but can sometimes cause

neurological damage. This emphasizes the importance of examining the entire spine.

2. Many spinal injury patients suffer from additional trauma, such as head, thoracic, or abdominal injuries, which can complicate treatment priorities.

3. Pain from other injuries may overshadow or mask spinal pain, delaying diagnosis.

Effects of Spinal Cord Injury on the Autonomic Nervous System

The autonomic nervous system (ANS) is heavily impacted by SCI, especially in injuries above the upper thoracic vertebrae, which disrupt both sympathetic and parasympathetic functions. The severity of dysfunction correlates with the level and extent of the injury.

Direct Effects

Cardiovascular: In cases of complete quadriplegia, loss of sympathetic tone leads to systemic vasodilation, resulting in hypotension (neurogenic shock). The absence of compensatory tachycardia or vasoconstriction due to sympathetic denervation means the body cannot counteract the drop in blood pressure. This can also cause bradycardia due to unopposed parasympathetic activity.

Gastrointestinal: A paralytic ileus often develops post-injury, typically resolving within 3-10 days. Sphincter paralysis and reduced abdominal wall muscle function can lead to complications such as aspiration or difficulty clearing the airway.

Urinary: In the acute phase, SCI can cause urinary retention due to bladder denervation and spinal shock. Inserting a catheter prevents over-distension and aids in monitoring urine output.

Thermoregulatory: Following a cervical or upper thoracic injury, the inability to regulate body temperature occurs due to loss of sympathetic control, resulting in difficulty maintaining heat in cold conditions and loss of sweating in warm environments.

Pre-Hospital Management

Extrication and Immobilization
Spinal immobilization in pre-hospital settings is challenging, especially when patients are trapped in vehicles, submerged, or in awkward positions. Emergency medical services (EMS) teams must use devices designed to provide in-line protection during extrication. Restlessness, possibly due to hypoxia, hypotension, or anxiety, can complicate the immobilization process. EMS personnel are trained to minimize movement, stabilize the spine, and transfer the patient for further care.

In-line Protection
When spinal injury is suspected, immediate in-line spinal protection is crucial, as more than 90% of suspected cervical spine injuries do not result in instability. Current guidelines recommend minimal handling, early manual immobilization, and quick transfer to definitive care. Although common spinal immobilization techniques have not been proven to significantly reduce neurological damage,

they remain standard in early trauma care to prevent movement and additional injury. However, pre-hospital devices, such as spine boards, should be removed promptly upon hospital arrival to avoid discomfort and reduce risks such as pressure sores or respiratory issues.

Initial Treatment

Primary Survey

Patients with suspected SCI are treated following standard trauma protocols, starting with a primary survey, resuscitation, secondary survey, and definitive management. Key considerations include:

Airway management: Particularly in cervical injuries, where passive regurgitation and aspiration of gastric contents can occur, airway protection is vital. A nasogastric tube may be required to prevent aspiration and ensure airway safety.

The causes of late-onset preeclampsia, which typically manifests after the 34th week of pregnancy, remain a subject of ongoing research. Although its pathophysiology is not fully understood, several factors contribute to its development. Primary among these is poor placental perfusion, which leads to endothelial dysfunction, activation of the maternal immune system, and systemic vascular resistance. This condition often correlates with pre existing maternal risk factors such as obesity, hypertension, and a history of preeclampsia in previous pregnancies, along with maternal age extremes (both young and advanced maternal age).

The roles of inflammatory cytokines, oxidative stress, and defective angiogenesis are also critical in the pathogenesis. These mechanisms contribute to the widespread vasoconstriction, endothelial injury, and subsequent hypertension observed in late-onset preeclampsia. Additionally, there is an association with abnormalities in the renin-angiotensin-aldosterone system, which further exacerbates the clinical manifestations.

Late-onset preeclampsia may present with less severe fetal growth restriction compared to early-onset forms, yet maternal and fetal morbidity remain significant. Clinical management of the condition focuses on blood pressure control, with the judicious use of antihypertensive agents such as labetalol, methyldopa, and nifedipine, as well as vigilant monitoring for signs of progression to severe preeclampsia or eclampsia.

Understanding the nuanced pathophysiology of late-onset preeclampsia is essential for improving early detection and outcomes. Ongoing research into biomarkers, genetic predispositions, and novel therapeutic interventions holds promise for more effective management in the future.

Mechanisms of Spinal Injuries:

1. Flexion-Rotation: This mechanism is responsible for unilateral facet dislocations or forward subluxation of the cervical spine. The force

applied causes one vertebra to rotate and slide forward relative to the vertebra below, resulting in displacement.

2. Vertebral Compression: This mechanism leads to burst fractures, where the intervertebral disc is driven into the vertebral body below. The disc may also be extruded into prevertebral tissues anteriorly or into the spinal canal posteriorly. The vertebral body may suffer comminution, with bone fragments extruding both anteriorly and posteriorly into the spinal canal.

3. Lateral Flexion: Injuries from lateral flexion can cause uncinate fractures, isolated pillar fractures, transverse process injuries, and lateral vertebral compression.

4. Distraction: Injuries from distraction result in significant disruption of the ligamentous structures and intervertebral discs. A hangman's fracture, which combines distraction with hyperextension, is a typical injury associated with this mechanism.

Cervical Spine Injuries:

1. C1 (Atlas) Fractures: Atlas fractures account for approximately 4% of cervical spine injuries. Hyperextension or compression mechanisms are the primary causes. Around 15-20% of these fractures are associated with C2 fractures, and 25% may involve lower cervical injuries. The Jefferson fracture, a blowout fracture of the atlas ring, is a notable example, along with isolated injuries to the posterior and anterior arches and lateral masses.

2. C2 (Axis) Fractures: Axis fractures account for 6% of cervical spine injuries, often in combination with C1 injuries. CT scans are used to detect odontoid subluxation. Three main types of odontoid fractures are:

Type 1: An avulsion of the odontoid tip, typically stable, representing 5-8% of odontoid fractures.

Type 2: A fracture at the base of the dens, generally unstable, and constitutes 55-70% of odontoid fractures. In children, this injury may be confused with a type 2 fracture due to the presence of the epiphysis.

Type 3: A fracture extending into the vertebral body, making up 30-35% of odontoid fractures.

Additionally, a hangman's fracture, a bilateral neural arch fracture of C2, occurs due to hyperextension and is associated with prevertebral soft tissue swelling, anterior subluxation of C2 on C3, and avulsion of the antero-inferior corner of C2.

3. C3–C7 Fractures: Fractures in this region are easily detected using CT scans. These fractures are considered unstable when:

Both anterior and posterior elements of the vertebrae are disrupted.

There is more than 3 mm overriding of the vertebral body above over the vertebral body below.

The angle between adjacent vertebrae exceeds 11 degrees.

The height of the anterior border of a vertebral body is less than two-thirds of the posterior border.

Thoracic Spine Injuries:
Hyperflexion is the primary cause of injuries in the thoracic spine, resulting in vertebral body wedging. Due to the rigidity of the thoracic cage, most thoracic spine injuries are stable, but internal stabilization may be needed if there is pronounced kyphosis.

Thoracolumbar Spine Injuries:
Injuries to the thoracolumbar spine account for 40% of vertebral fractures with neurological deficits. These are commonly caused by flexion or hyperflexion-rotation mechanisms. Plain films may reveal facet joint disruption, interspinal ligament damage, posterior bony fragments protruding into the spinal canal, and burst fractures at the vertebral body's superior surface. These fractures are typically unstable.

Lumbar Spine Injuries:
In the lumbar spine, the types of injuries observed are similar to those in the thoracolumbar region, with a focus on posterior distraction injuries of the vertebral arch. Specifically,

seatbelt injuries occur when a hyperflexion force is applied to a person wearing a lap-only seat belt. These injuries result from deceleration in high-speed incidents, such as head-on collisions or aircraft crashes.

Imaging and Diagnosis:

Plain films are typically the first-line imaging study. Key radiological findings include:

A vacant or empty appearance of the vertebral body on an AP view.

Discontinuity in the cortex of the pedicles or spinous processes on the AP view.

Fractures or dislocations, which may be subtle on lateral views.

CT and MRI are valuable for further detailing architectural disruptions. However, fractures in axial planes may be challenging to detect, as they often align parallel to the scanning plane. Three-dimensional reconstruction of multislice CT images has significantly improved spinal injury imaging.

Thoracolumbar fractures are often associated with concurrent intra-abdominal visceral injuries, which should be considered during diagnosis and treatment.

Specific Fractures:

1.   Chance   Fractures: Characterized by an oblique or horizontal splitting of the spinous process and neural arch, these fractures extend into the intervertebral disc, damaging it.

2. Horizontal Fissure Fractures: Similar to Chance fractures but with a horizontal fracture line that extends through the vertebral body's anterior aspect.

3. Smith Fractures: These fractures spare the posterior spinous process but involve the superior articular processes and a small posterior fragment. Posterior ligament disruption is a characteristic feature.

Spinal Shock vs. Neurogenic Shock:

Spinal shock is often confused with neurogenic shock, but they are distinct entities. Spinal shock refers to the cessation of cord activity below the injury level, with the cord unable to function due to the absence of descending facilitatory impulses. Recovery is indicated by the return of reflexes, such as the Babinski response.

Spinal Cord Injuries:

Primary spinal cord injuries result from trauma-induced damage directly to the spinal cord, while secondary injuries involve subsequent damage caused by factors like hypotension or hypoxia.

Transverse Cord Syndrome involves complete transverse damage to the spinal cord, resulting in total paralysis, anesthesia, and analgesia below the injury site. Partial recovery may occur in incomplete cases.

Central Cervical Cord Syndrome typically occurs from hyperextension injuries and is seen in older individuals with cervical spondylosis. It causes weakness in both upper and lower limbs, with more significant weakness in the upper limbs.

Anterior Cervical Cord Syndrome involves injury to the anterior spinal cord, leading to motor paralysis, loss of pain and temperature sensation, but preservation of joint position, vibration sense, and fine touch.

Brown-Séquard Syndrome is a functional cord hemisection lesion with ipsilateral motor impairment and loss of light touch, vibration, and joint position sense, while contralateral loss of pain and temperature sensation occurs.

Posterior Cord Syndrome involves damage to the dorsal columns, causing disruptions to proprioception, vibration, and fine touch sensation.

Spinal Cord Concussion refers to temporary cessation of spinal cord function, usually recovering within 48 hours, and involves no significant anatomical injury.

Chapter 8 (C)
Facial Trauma Assessment and Management in the Emergency Department (ED)

This chapter focuses on the evaluation and management of facial injuries in the Emergency Department (ED). It provides a comprehensive overview of facial trauma, emphasizing the importance of immediate care, proper assessment, and strategies for managing complex cases. Eye and dental injuries are discussed in other sections of this book.

Prevalence and Causes of Facial Injuries

Facial trauma is most commonly observed in young males, with contributing factors such as alcohol or drug intoxication. The causes of facial injuries vary globally, with road accidents, interpersonal violence, falls, and sports injuries being prevalent among adults. In the developing world, road trauma is increasingly frequent, while developed nations have seen a reduction due to improved road safety measures. Additionally, the aging population in developed countries has led to an increase in falls among the elderly. Intimate partner violence is another significant cause, particularly affecting women.

Anatomy and Functions of the Face

The face consists of a bony structure suspended beneath the base of the anterior and middle cranial fossae. It is supported by layers of muscles, including the superficial muscles of facial expression, deep muscles of mastication, and those of the tongue and oropharynx. Key organs include the eyes, salivary and lacrimal glands, as well as parts of the gastrointestinal and respiratory systems. The face plays vital roles in eating, drinking, breathing, and sensory functions (sight, hearing, smell, taste, and touch). Social functions such as facial expression, speech, and identification are critical to human interaction.

The primary goal of managing facial trauma is to restore the facial structure as close to its normal appearance and function as possible, as facial injuries may impact both physical appearance and psychological well-being.

Associated Injuries

Facial trauma is often associated with other life-threatening injuries. The likelihood of such injuries depends on the force of the trauma and the severity of the facial injury. High-energy impacts, such as those from motor vehicle crashes, can lead to fractures of the frontal bone or symphysis mandible, and may also cause blunt cerebrovascular injury. On the other hand, low-energy injuries, such as a punch to the face, are less likely to result in serious injuries beyond the face itself.

In the elderly, even minor falls can lead to complex, multi-system trauma due to age-related frailty, comorbidities, and polypharmacy.

History and Primary Survey

For all trauma patients, understanding the mechanism of injury is critical for proper risk stratification and management. It is important to inquire sensitively about intimate partner violence and document any use of anticoagulants or antiplatelet medications.

The primary survey should be conducted as usual, ensuring life-threatening injuries are identified and managed before focusing on the facial injury. If the facial trauma is life-threatening, it is typically due to airway obstruction or uncontrolled hemorrhage.

Airway Management

Managing the airway in facial trauma presents significant challenges, particularly when the trauma threatens the airway due to blood, swelling, or debris such as teeth or bone fragments. For less severe trauma, patients may be able to manage their own airway in a comfortable position, but more severe cases often require supine positioning and assistance.

In trauma centers, an experienced trauma team should manage the airway, utilizing techniques like jaw thrusts and suction. In cases of unstable fractures, anterior traction may be necessary to open the airway and reduce bleeding. In severe cases, rapid sequence induction and possible surgical airway placement may be required.

Breathing and Circulation

Assessment of breathing focuses on other injuries or

potential lung damage due to aspirated blood or foreign objects like teeth. Circulation should be closely monitored, as 5% of midface fractures can cause life-threatening hemorrhage. Most bleeding can be controlled with nasal packing, direct pressure, and topical agents such as tranexamic acid. In more severe cases, packing the entire pharynx may be necessary.

It is important to be cautious when managing patients with facial fractures, as these injuries are often associated with base-of-skull fractures. Careful attention must be paid during nasal packing to avoid entering the cranial cavity.

Secondary Survey

During the secondary survey, the physician should look for asymmetry, abnormal contours, or tenderness on palpation of bony structures. Patients should be asked to assess their own dental integrity by feeling their teeth and checking occlusion. Nerve function, including that of the trigeminal nerve (responsible for sensory input to the face) and the facial nerve (responsible for facial expression), must also be evaluated.

Imaging and Diagnostics

Computed tomography (CT) is the primary imaging technique for assessing facial injuries due to its ability to capture detailed images. The orthopantomogram (OPG) is still useful for dental surgeons when planning treatments. Point-of-care ultrasound is gaining a role in assessing the eye when there is significant swelling, but it is avoided if an open globe injury is suspected.

Physical Examination for Specific Injuries

The physical examination should focus on detecting specific injuries associated with facial trauma. For instance, eye injuries may involve enophthalmos (sunken eye), exophthalmos (bulging eye), or visual disturbances such as diplopia (double vision). Mandibular fractures may result in malocclusion or pain while biting. For nasal injuries, septal hematomas and cerebrospinal fluid leakage should be considered. Careful inspection of the oral cavity and ear is also critical for detecting fractures or foreign body injuries.

Conclusion

Facial trauma presents a complex set of challenges that require careful, systematic assessment and management. While restoring normal anatomy is essential, functional outcomes—such as preserving sensory and motor functions—are equally important. Early identification and management of associated injuries are key to improving outcomes for these patients.

Key Takeaways:

1. Facial trauma often occurs as part of a broader set of injuries, including those resulting from violence, sports accidents, and road trauma.

2. Airway and hemorrhage management are primary concerns in the initial stages of treatment.

3. Imaging tools such as CT and OPG play a crucial role in diagnosing facial fractures.

4.   Understanding   the relationship between structure and function is essential to managing facial injuries, as cosmetic outcomes cannot be separated from functional recovery.

5.   Prompt,   effective management of associated injuries significantly improves patient outcomes.

Disposition of Facial Injuries:

Most facial wounds can be effectively treated in the emergency department (ED) with attention to key anatomical landmarks (e.g., the vermilion border in lip lacerations). It is essential to assess for involvement of underlying structures such as the parotid duct in cheek lacerations or the tarsal plates and lacrimal apparatus in eyelid injuries. Surgical debridement is generally avoided to preserve cosmesis, and antibiotics are typically not required, though thorough cleaning is critical, particularly in dirty injuries or those caused by bites.

Facial fractures are usually managed after swelling

subsides, once more severe injuries are addressed. Isolated facial fractures often allow for discharge from the ED with a scheduled surgical outpatient follow-up unless complications like pain, bleeding, or swelling require admission.

Proper documentation of examination findings and treatment is crucial, especially in assault cases, as it supports forensic evidence.

Specific Facial Injuries:

1. Soft Tissue Injuries: Soft tissue injuries to the face (abrasions, contusions, lacerations, avulsions, burns) aim to preserve both function and appearance. The decision to repair wounds in the ED depends on the severity and nature of the injury. Delayed wound closure is considered for cases with more urgent injuries, severe crush trauma, foreign bodies, significant contamination, or underlying fractures. Such wounds should be irrigated, hemostasis achieved, and covered with saline-soaked gauze before referral to a specialist.

Certain facial injuries, such as ocular trauma, significant eyelid injuries, parotid gland or duct injuries, and facial nerve damage, require surgical intervention and are best managed in the operating room. Specialized areas like the lips, perioral region, nose, ears, and eyes require extra consideration due to their complex anatomy. For example, the eyebrow should not be shaved, and subperichondrial hematomas of the ear require drainage within 7-10 days to prevent "cauliflower ear."

Wounds treated in the ED must undergo meticulous cleansing, preferably using pulsatile saline irrigation. Abrasions with embedded dirt or foreign bodies require thorough scrubbing to avoid dermal tattooing. Multi-layer repairs are advisable for deeper wounds, particularly those involving subcutaneous structures, to minimize deep tissue infections and improve cosmetic results.

Vision loss from blunt facial trauma may result from direct injury to the eye, optic nerve, or due to increased intraocular pressure, such as in orbital compartment syndrome (OCS). OCS, although rare, requires timely intervention through lateral canthotomy and inferior cantholysis to relieve pressure.

2. Facial Fractures: Facial skeletal fractures typically disperse force to protect the skull and brain. The mandible and maxilla require more force to fracture compared to the nasal bones. Diagnosing facial fractures involves inspection, palpation, and radiographic assessment. Most fractures, other than non-displaced nasal, zygomatic, or maxillary fractures, require prompt maxillofacial surgical evaluation. Initial management often includes head elevation and ice application.

Mandible Fractures: The mandible's horseshoe shape leads to fractures at certain vulnerable points. Common fracture sites include the condylar neck, angle, and body near the molars. Treatment typically involves internal fixation, and complications may include numbness, delayed healing, infection, or misalignment of teeth. Although evidence for prophylactic antibiotics is limited, they are commonly administered before surgery.

Zygomatic Fractures: Isolated fractures of the zygomatic arch are rare, often part of larger zygomatic complex fractures. Surgical reduction is necessary for cosmetic restoration and to restore normal mandibular movement.

Zygomatic Complex (Tripod) Fractures: Blunt trauma to the zygoma can lead to a tripod fracture, involving fractures at multiple suture lines (zygomaticofrontal, zygomaticotemporal, and zygomaticomaxillary). These fractures often affect the lateral wall of the maxillary sinus and orbital floor. Up to 20% of these fractures are associated with ocular injuries.

Orbital Fractures: Orbital floor fractures, often part of zygomaticomaxillary fractures, or isolated orbital blowout fractures, can result in herniation of orbital contents into the maxillary sinus. These fractures require CT scans for full evaluation, and any signs of optic nerve compression call for immediate surgical intervention. All orbital fractures should be referred for specialized care.

Maxillary Fractures: Maxillary fractures include fractures of the alveolar ridge, anterolateral maxillary sinus wall, and Le Fort fractures. These fractures often occur in combination. Le Fort fractures are classified into three types: I (horizontal maxillary fracture), II (pyramidal fracture), and III (craniofacial disjunction). Urgent intervention is needed for Le Fort II and III fractures to prevent airway obstruction and control bleeding. These injuries may also lead to cerebrospinal fluid (CSF) leakage, necessitating a thorough eye examination.

Nasal Fractures: Nasal fractures are common and often diagnosed clinically, as X-rays are usually unnecessary. The main concerns are controlling bleeding and excluding septal hematoma. Severe displacement may require early reduction in the ED, but most fractures can be reduced within 7-10 days.

Nasoethmoidal Fractures: These complex fractures involve the nose and medial orbital structures, often causing widening of the intercanthal distance or changes to the palpebral fissures. Referral is necessary due to the risk of persistent epistaxis and CSF rhinorrhoea.

Temporomandibular Joint (TMJ) Injuries: TMJ injuries often result from trauma to the temporal bone and can affect the middle and inner ear structures. Dislocation commonly occurs from excessive mouth opening and is diagnosed by X-ray. Successful relocation can be achieved with gentle pressure and manipulation. Post-reduction care includes analgesia and diet modifications, along with advice to avoid wide mouth opening.

3. Penetrating Facial Injuries: Penetrating injuries such as gunshot wounds, stabbings, and impaling objects may cause severe tissue and bone damage, though they are rarely fatal. The severity of these injuries depends on factors like projectile mass, velocity, and the density of the affected tissue. Airway management is crucial in gunshot wounds, as these injuries can lead to rapid respiratory failure. Shotgun and stab wounds are less likely to cause airway obstruction but still pose risks due to vascular injury or swelling, particularly when the injury affects the mandible.

Chapter 8 (D)
Abdominal trauma

Abdominal injuries account for approximately 10% of trauma-related deaths. These injuries often remain undiagnosed at first, as they are not immediately visible, and common diagnostic tools like plain radiography have limited sensitivity in detecting intra-abdominal bleeding or damage to solid organs. Furthermore, symptoms such as blood loss might be overlooked in favor of more apparent injuries, making abdominal trauma a leading cause of preventable death in trauma patients. Thus, a high level of suspicion is necessary to prevent morbidity and mortality associated with these injuries.

A structured approach to managing patients with multiple injuries should prioritize the identification of abdominal trauma. The primary goals of initial care are to assess whether an abdominal injury exists, determine if surgical intervention is needed, and decide on the timing of any necessary procedures. An experienced clinician should oversee this process as early as possible, ideally with the trauma surgeon involved from the outset, especially during the initial resuscitation phase.

The steps of primary and secondary surveys, along with history-taking, physical examination, and specific investigations, are crucial for managing trauma patients.

Primary and Secondary Surveys

During the primary survey, assessing circulation may help identify potential intra-abdominal hemorrhage, especially in unstable patients who require ongoing fluid resuscitation without any apparent external bleeding. Comprehensive abdominal examination, including the back, rectum, and vagina, is essential. Any examination should be thorough, ensuring that all relevant regions are assessed.

History

The mechanism of injury can provide significant insight into the likelihood of substantial intra-abdominal trauma. Emergency responders can offer valuable details about the incident. Trauma often affects multiple body areas, and substantial abdominal injuries may occur even when no external abdominal trauma is evident. A focused history should include the AMPLE acronym: Allergies, Medications, Past medical history, Last eaten or drank, and Events surrounding the trauma incident.

Abdominal Examination

Penetrating injuries are typically obvious, while blunt trauma, which is more common, is harder to detect clinically. Bruising and abrasions may suggest internal abdominal injury, particularly to the spleen or liver, which are the most frequently injured organs. The patterns of injury differ between blunt and penetrating trauma. Specific signs, such as marks from lap seat belts, may be associated with particular fractures or organ injuries. Palpation can reveal localized tenderness or generalized discomfort, which may indicate peritonitis or abdominal injury, but it may not always identify retroperitoneal injuries. Auscultation is rarely helpful, but the absence of bowel sounds can raise concern for intra-abdominal trauma.

For a comprehensive assessment, it is important to examine the back, buttocks, and perineum, especially in obese patients where skin folds may hide penetrating injuries. Rectal and vaginal exams can uncover signs of bleeding or other significant findings, such as tamponade or a pregnant uterus, in unconscious patients.

Key Risk Factors for Abdominal Injury

Several factors can increase the risk of intra-abdominal trauma, including high-speed vehicle collisions, pedestrian impacts, falls from significant heights, hypotension, and major chest or pelvic injuries. Box 3.5.1 outlines other relevant risk factors.

Essentials for Diagnosis and Management

1. Abdominal injuries contribute to approximately 10% of trauma deaths.

2. These injuries may not be immediately apparent due to overshadowing external or orthopedic injuries, requiring a heightened index of suspicion.

3. Early detection is crucial to prevent preventable morbidity and mortality.

4. Computed tomography (CT) is useful for organ-specific diagnosis, but patient stability is necessary for safe transport.

5. Focused Assessment with Sonography for Trauma (FAST) can aid in evaluating suspected abdominal injuries, though it has limitations.

6. Abdominal trauma often coexists with other injuries, and prompt involvement of a senior trauma surgeon can improve evaluation and management.

Investigations

Initial trauma management includes obtaining blood samples for complete blood count (CBC), electrolytes, blood glucose, cross-matching, and blood gas analysis, in addition to radiologic imaging. However, traditional abdominal radiography has limited utility. Gunshot and stab wounds require immediate assessment, often involving laparotomy. If surgery is not immediately necessary, further imaging such as ultrasound or CT scans can help guide management.

Unstable patients, where immediate intervention is

required, should be transferred to surgery without delay. Stable patients can undergo further investigation to guide their treatment plan. For those with suspected abdominal trauma, but who cannot be fully assessed clinically—such as patients with head, chest, or spinal injuries, or those under sedation—additional imaging techniques like ultrasound and CT are valuable tools. Each method has its advantages and limitations, but when combined, they offer a comprehensive assessment.

Abdominal CT vs. Ultrasound

CT provides detailed anatomic images and can visualize the retroperitoneum and adjacent areas such as the chest and pelvis. Its limitations include radiation exposure, potential contrast reactions, and the need to transport unstable patients to the scanner. CT is typically reserved for stable patients who can tolerate transfer.

On the other hand, ultrasound is a rapid, non-invasive, and bedside method that can be used repeatedly, making it especially useful in unstable patients. In experienced hands, ultrasound can provide critical information, including the detection of free fluid, blood, or gas, and can assess cardiac function. However, it requires skilled operators, and its accuracy in identifying specific injuries, such as hollow organ damage, is less reliable than CT.

Interventional Radiology

The increasing role of interventional radiology provides another option for managing unstable patients with retroperitoneal or pelvic bleeding. Some centers now use hybrid suites, combining CT, interventional radiology, and operating theater capabilities, to streamline patient care.

Focused Assessment with Sonography in Trauma (FAST)

Focused abdominal ultrasound, performed at the bedside, offers a rapid, non-invasive means of identifying intraperitoneal injury in trauma patients. With high sensitivity and specificity, FAST is an invaluable tool in evaluating patients with suspected intra-abdominal trauma. Additionally, it can detect other complications such as hemopericardium or hemothorax. While FAST is a highly effective diagnostic tool, its limitations include operator dependency and the inability to detect some injuries, such as those involving the diaphragm or hollow organs.

Chapter 8 (E)
Chest trauma

Essentials:

1. The initial management of patients with chest trauma involves securing oxygenation, providing ventilatory support if necessary, performing pleural and pericardial decompression when appropriate, supporting circulation, ensuring effective pain relief, and obtaining early imaging to identify potentially life-threatening injuries.

2. Fewer than 10% of patients with blunt chest trauma require surgical intervention.

3. Supine chest radiographs may not reliably rule out conditions such as hemothorax, pneumothorax, aortic injury,

diaphragmatic rupture, cardiac tamponade, or fractures of the ribs, sternum, thoracic spine, and scapula.

4. Multislice computed tomography (CT) with intravenous contrast is the gold standard for screening and diagnosing thoracic injuries. Ultrasound can help detect hemothorax, pneumothorax, pulmonary contusion, cardiac tamponade, and diaphragmatic injury.

5. Aseptic, percutaneous digital identification of the pleural space is the crucial first step in pleural decompression, followed by chest tube insertion. Needle thoracocentesis is generally ineffective in decompressing the chest in unstable patients.

6. Pleural decompression and chest tube placement during resuscitation are associated with a low risk of complications.

7. Resuscitative thoracotomy plays an important role in shocked patients who show evidence of cardiac tamponade on ultrasound.

8. Non-invasive ventilation may help prevent complications associated with mechanical ventilation in certain patients with flail chest and pulmonary contusion.

Introduction

Incidence

Thoracic trauma accounts for approximately 25% of all trauma-related fatalities and contributes to an additional 25% of trauma cases. In regions such as Australasia and the United Kingdom, blunt trauma causes 90-95% of chest injuries.

Principles of Initial Management

The initial management of thoracic trauma focuses on key priorities: ensuring oxygenation, providing ventilatory support if necessary, performing pleural and pericardial decompression when indicated, circulatory support, pain management, and early imaging to identify evolving life-threatening injuries. The majority of patients with chest trauma can be treated without surgery, with fewer than 10% of blunt trauma cases requiring thoracotomy. The remaining cases primarily need supportive care, such as pleural decompression and drainage.

Resuscitation, in particular, is often suboptimal. Delays or inadequacies in ventilatory support, shock management, arterial blood gas monitoring, pleural decompression, and definitive imaging can lead to preventable morbidity and mortality. Immediate life-threatening injuries, such as flail chest, pulmonary contusion, thoracic aortic transection, pneumothorax, hemothorax, pericardial tamponade, and ruptured diaphragm, may not be immediately apparent. These conditions should be actively ruled out, as routine supine chest X-rays are not sufficient for this purpose. Multi-slice CT with contrast is the gold standard for screening high-risk patients, though life-saving procedures should take priority. Ultrasound can be used to quickly identify conditions like cardiac tamponade and hemothorax.

Oxygenation

Hypoxia may not be present at the initial assessment of chest trauma but can develop as the injuries progress. Supplemental oxygen should be administered to address mild desaturation, with adjustments made based on clinical response. In more severe cases, higher concentrations of oxygen can be delivered using positive airway pressure or invasive ventilation techniques, such as continuous positive airway pressure (CPAP) or expiratory positive airway pressure (EPAP). Modifying the inspiratory/expiratory (I/E) ratio in mechanically ventilated patients with severe hypoxia may also provide benefits. However, advanced techniques such as independent lung ventilation, inhaled nitric oxide, and extracorporeal membrane oxygenation have unproven benefits during initial resuscitation.

Pulmonary Support

Pain, fatigue from increased work of breathing, and opiate analgesia can lead to hypoventilation. Patients, particularly the elderly or those with pre-existing chest wall compliance issues, may be at higher risk.

Non-Invasive Ventilation (NIV)

In cases of pulmonary contusions and high oxygen demand, patients may not need intubation and can be effectively managed with non-invasive ventilation (NIV). NIV has been shown to reduce the risk of nosocomial infections, which are common with mechanical ventilation.

Mechanical Ventilation

NIV may be contraindicated in trauma patients requiring full spinal precautions, those with impaired consciousness, or those with facial injuries. For patients with pulmonary contusions and poor lung compliance, mechanical ventilation should be performed using low tidal volumes and low inspiratory pressures to minimize barotrauma and secondary lung injury.

Fluid Resuscitation

Evidence supports the use of "permissive hypotension" in penetrating torso injuries before surgical intervention. This approach can improve survival, reduce the need for blood products, and minimize coagulopathy. However, it is uncertain whether this strategy is beneficial in hypotensive blunt trauma. Once hemorrhage is controlled, optimizing fluid therapy to enhance cardiac output and oxygen delivery may improve survival. Conservative fluid management is particularly important in patients with pulmonary contusion to avoid increasing extravascular lung water. However, under-resuscitation can worsen organ dysfunction, and invasive monitoring may be necessary to guide fluid replacement.

Analgesia

Effective pain management is essential to reduce hypoventilation and facilitate respiratory functions, such as coughing and physiotherapy, to prevent atelectasis and consolidation. Oral analgesics are sufficient for managing single rib fractures, but more extensive pain control, such as parenteral narcotics or intercostal nerve blocks, is required for multiple rib fractures. Advanced regional nerve blocks, like epidural or paravertebral blocks, offer greater efficacy but carry a higher risk of complications.

Indications for Emergency Thoracotomy

While over 90% of chest trauma patients can be managed non-surgically, some cases require surgical intervention, including:

Cardiac tamponade

Acute deterioration, such as cardiac arrest from penetrating truncal trauma

Thoracic outlet vascular injury

Traumatic chest wall loss

Massive or persistent hemothorax

Mediastinal or oesophageal injury

Tracheal or bronchial injury

Resuscitative thoracotomy, typically performed with the arms in a cruciform position, provides access to the chest for procedures like pericardial decompression, cardiac massage, and vascular control. Survival rates for penetrating trauma are higher when resuscitative thoracotomy is performed within 10 minutes of arrest.

Focused assessment with sonography in trauma (FAST) can help identify cardiac tamponade. Early ultrasonography and prompt repair of injuries can improve survival, particularly in patients with severe hypotension or those who are in .

Thoracic Injuries

Fractured Ribs

Rib fractures are common and can lead to pain, which impairs ventilation and promotes atelectasis. Rib fractures may be associated with injuries to underlying structures like the lungs, pleura, or intercostal vessels. Fractures of the lower ribs may indicate splenic or hepatic injuries, while fractures of posterior ribs can be associated with renal injuries. Although first- and second-rib fractures were once thought to indicate thoracic aortic injury, this association is now questioned. Rib fractures are often diagnosed clinically, as chest X-rays may not detect up to 50% of fractures. Pain management is key to preventing complications like atelectasis, and interventions like patient-controlled narcotics, local anesthetic blocks, and incentive spirometry are commonly used.

Fractured Sternum

Sternal fractures, diagnosed via CT scan or X-ray, often accompany intrathoracic injuries such as myocardial damage. In regions with lower seat belt usage, sternal fractures are more common due to impacts against the steering wheel, whereas in areas with higher seat belt use, fractures typically occur due to the restraining belt. For isolated sternal fractures, brief hospitalization for pain management is usually sufficient unless cardiac injury is suspected.

Vertebral and Spinal Cord Injury

Assessing spinal stability is crucial before sitting the patient up, to avoid exacerbating ventilation/perfusion mismatch. Spinal injuries are common but often overlooked, especially in patients requiring ventilation. Stability must be evaluated and addressed as part of the routine work-up for chest trauma patients.

Flail Chest

Flail chest occurs when the chest wall is fractured in at least two places, resulting in paradoxical movement of the affected area. This condition often leads to ventilation issues, worsened by pain and pulmonary contusion. Treatment focuses on maintaining oxygenation, ventilation, and fluid balance, with analgesia through intercostal nerve blocks or epidural analgesia. Patients with significant flail chest often require respiratory support to ensure adequate ventilation.

Myocardial Contusion

Myocardial contusion, though relatively common, seldom leads to significant complications. Cardiac failure and hypotension are rare outcomes associated with this condition. While the electrocardiogram (ECG) is commonly employed to predict myocardial contusion, it is not highly specific and is not particularly effective at evaluating the right ventricle—the region most often affected. Elevations in cardiac enzymes may occur but are not reliable indicators of injury. Echocardiography may reveal abnormal wall motion or dyskinesis in the affected ventricular area. Magnetic Resonance Imaging (MRI) provides a more sensitive and specific method of diagnosis, though it requires specialized resources and expertise. For patients with acute ECG abnormalities or conduction disturbances, hospitalization and monitoring for potential arrhythmias are recommended.

Myocardial Laceration and Cardiac Tamponade

Penetrating injuries to the chest, particularly precordial wounds, may result in myocardial lacerations. Bedside sonography is useful for detecting myocardial injury and pericardial fluid accumulation. Patients presenting with signs of pericardial tamponade (such as hypotension, muffled heart sounds, and jugular venous distention) need prompt surgical intervention. In cases where patients deteriorate into cardiac arrest despite showing signs of life prior to or upon arrival at the hospital, resuscitative thoracotomy should be considered. This procedure is typically reserved for patients with a potential for survival. The prognosis is extremely poor for patients without initial signs of life, particularly in blunt trauma cases, with survival rates under 2%. However, survival is more common in penetrating injuries. External cardiac massage for more than 9 minutes is generally futile for these patients.

Tension Pneumopericardium

Tension pneumopericardium, though far less common than tension pneumothorax, typically results from a 'one-way valve' mechanism, especially after the onset of positive-pressure ventilation. It presents with symptoms like elevated central venous pressure and hypotension, responding favorably to urgent pericardial decompression.

Thoracic Aortic Transection

Thoracic aortic transection has a very high mortality rate, with 85% of patients dying before reaching the hospital. This injury is often caused by high deceleration forces, which result in shearing forces that tear the aorta, particularly at the ligamentum . Immediate diagnosis and treatment are critical, as up to 50% of patients with incomplete aortic transections may die within 48 hours without surgical intervention. Chest x-rays showing mediastinal widening are a common finding, but they are not sufficiently specific for aortic injury. In high-risk trauma patients, contrast-enhanced chest CT scans should be used to exclude aortic injury. Treatment typically focuses on reducing blood pressure to prevent further shearing and using a stent for vascular repair. Open surgery is less common due to high mortality rates, with endovascular stent placement being the preferred method.

Esophageal Perforation

Blunt chest trauma rarely causes esophageal rupture, which commonly occurs in the lower third of the esophagus. This may be due to a forced Valsalva maneuver, leading to mediastinitis. Retrosternal pain is a typical symptom, and mediastinal air may be visible on chest radiographs. CT scans with a Gastrografin swallow are the preferred diagnostic methods. Gunshot wounds that traverse the truncal midline tend to involve mediastinal and spinal structures and have a higher mortality rate. Early identification of esophageal injury is essential to reduce morbidity and mortality in these cases.

Future Considerations

Advancements in healthcare systems, imaging technologies, and diagnostic methods are expected to facilitate earlier detection and treatment of chest trauma. Improved ultrasound use is emerging for chest trauma assessment, and conservative management for occult pneumothoraces is gaining traction, though further research is needed to confirm its safety. The increasing use of non-invasive ventilation (NIV) and operative rib fixation for managing flail chest injuries is also noteworthy.

Conclusion

The severity of chest trauma may not always be immediately evident, as injuries can evolve over time. Most patients with severe blunt thoracic trauma require supportive care, including chest decompression and drainage. Ventilatory or respiratory compromise dictates the need for urgent chest decompression. Special attention should be given to patients with underlying airway diseases or diminished lung compliance, especially the elderly. Delayed or inadequate management of shock, respiratory distress, arterial blood gas monitoring, pleural decompression, and diagnostic imaging remain areas for improvement in emergency care.

Chapter 8 (F)
Limb trauma

Introduction

Limb injuries are among the most common causes of trauma-related visits to emergency departments (EDs) and are a significant source of long-term disability. These injuries can range from mild and inconsequential to life-threatening and severely debilitating. They often involve not only soft tissues and bones but also neurovascular structures. While some injuries may occur in isolation, others can involve multiple anatomical structures, especially in cases of severe trauma.

A holistic approach is essential in the management of limb injuries, particularly in patients with major trauma. The primary goal should be to treat the patient as a whole, rather than focusing on individual injuries or fractures. A comprehensive primary survey should be conducted for all patients, with life-threatening conditions addressed as the highest priority. Orthopedic injuries, including fractures, should be evaluated during the secondary survey. However, significant bleeding, particularly from open fractures like femoral fractures, may necessitate attention during the primary survey as part of circulatory assessment.

Open fractures and crush injuries are associated with specific complications, such as excessive bleeding, crush syndrome, hyperkalemia, and sepsis. Early intervention to control hemorrhage and administer appropriate antibiotics is crucial. Other potential complications include compartment syndrome and fat embolism syndrome, which will be discussed in detail later.

In the context of trauma, the immediate life-threatening concern associated with fractures is hemorrhagic shock. Limb trauma can also complicate trauma resuscitation by limiting access to veins for intravenous (IV) lines. Injured or deformed limbs should be avoided when placing IV lines, and in cases with multiple limb injuries, early central venous access may be required. Blood loss estimates include:

1200 to 1500 mL for femoral fractures

500 to 1000 mL for tibial fractures

500 mL for humeral fractures

The main objectives in managing multiple trauma patients are hemorrhage control and limb preservation. Ultimately, the goal of limb trauma care is to restore the patient to full, pain-free functionality with a focus on achieving good cosmetic outcomes. Upper limbs are essential for communication and interaction with the environment, while lower limbs serve primarily for independent ambulation. Rehabilitation is a key part of the recovery process and should involve early engagement with physiotherapists and occupational therapists.

Fractures

A fracture involves a break in bone continuity, which often includes damage to the surrounding soft tissues. The importance of the soft tissue component is often underestimated. For example, tense or pale skin over a closed fracture requires urgent reduction, even before imaging is performed. Skin that is ischemic, such as over the anterior tibia, is highly prone to necrosis and poorly responds to grafting, which can lead to amputation in severe cases.

Patients being transferred should have splints removed and the underlying tissues thoroughly assessed. No splint should remain in place for more than 8 hours without reassessment. Discharged patients must be given clear instructions for follow-up if they experience worsening pain, tightness under casts or splints, or numbness and pain distal to the fracture. Early follow-up is essential.

Fractures with intact overlying skin are classified as closed fractures, while open fractures are exposed to the environment. Open fractures are further categorized into:

Grade I: A wound less than 1 cm, clean

Grade II: A wound greater than 1 cm without extensive soft tissue damage

Grade III: Severe fractures with significant soft tissue damage, extensive contamination, or arterial injury

The risk of complications from fractures is higher in certain populations, including the elderly, immunocompromised individuals, alcoholics, and patients with peripheral vascular disease. High-risk trauma mechanisms include falls from a height greater than 3 meters, as well as injuries sustained by pedestrians, motorcyclists, or high-speed motorists. Severely head-injured patients are at greater risk of complications, particularly due to coagulopathy, which can increase bleeding from fractures. In addition, altered consciousness from head injury or sedation can complicate the clinical assessment of limb trauma.

Associated Injuries

1. Vascular Injury

Arterial injuries in limb trauma represent a serious and potentially life-threatening concern. Prolonged ischemia (more than 4-6 hours) can lead to irreversible tissue damage. It is essential to assess peripheral circulation and compare pulses on both sides. When there is active hemorrhage from a limb injury, direct pressure or hemostatic dressings should be applied. If bleeding persists, a tourniquet may be needed temporarily to control hemorrhage until definitive care can be provided.

The presence of a distal pulse does not rule out arterial injury, which may be incomplete.

Other signs that suggest vascular injury include limb deformity, dislocation, brisk bleeding, reduced pulses, and expanding hematoma. Common sites of arterial injury include:
Brachial artery (upper limb)
Popliteal artery (knee region)
Deep femoral artery (femoral region)
Anterior tibial artery (lower leg)
Computed tomography angiography (CTA) has largely replaced conventional angiography as the preferred diagnostic tool for suspected vascular injuries. Early consultation with a vascular surgeon is recommended when vascular injuries are suspected.

2. Nerve Injury

Nerve damage can occur due to direct lacerations by foreign bodies or fracture fragments, or from crushing, bruising, or stretching of nerves. It is important to rule out ischemia as a cause of neurological deficits. Penetrating trauma-related nerve injuries should be explored surgically. Nerve injuries can be classified as follows:

Neuropraxia: Temporary loss of nerve function, often from crushing or stretching. Full recovery typically occurs within 8 weeks.

Axonotmesis: Severe nerve injury with an intact nerve sheath. Regeneration may occur over several months.

Neurotmesis: Complete nerve division, requiring surgical repair. Spontaneous regeneration is unlikely.

Key nerve injury presentations include:

Wrist drop (radial nerve injury)

Foot drop (peroneal nerve injury)

Shoulder numbness/weakness (axillary nerve injury)

Sciatic nerve injury (posterior hip dislocation)

Median/ulnar nerve injury (wrist and forearm fractures)

Presentation

1. History and Examination

The history of limb trauma should be communicated using the MIST format upon arrival at the hospital:

Mechanism of injury

Injuries identified or suspected, including blood loss estimates, limb deformity, or amputation

Symptoms and signs, particularly vital signs, limb weakness or numbness, and pale or pulseless limbs

Treatments commenced and responses, including details of splints used

A thorough history should also include the patient's normal health status, medications, allergies, tetanus prophylaxis, and fasting state. The primary survey should be completed first, followed by a detailed secondary survey. Splints should be removed during trauma assessment, especially for patients transferred from other hospitals.

2. Assessment

The limb assessment includes:

Inspection for deformities, bruising, open fractures, bleeding, or pressure-induced skin changes, with comparison to the uninjured limb.

Palpation for pain, crepitus, or deformity.

Active and passive movement testing. Full active movement

in joints typically excludes dislocations.

Vascular assessment includes checking pulses and capillary refill.

Neurological assessment includes motor function and sensory testing, with two-point discrimination being the most accurate indicator of sensory function.

In cases of dislocated elbows or knees, vascular injury should be suspected, regardless of normal peripheral vascular examination findings.

Abnormal findings that suggest vascular injury include absent or reduced pulses, prolonged capillary refill, pale extremities, and expanding hematomas.

The Role of Splints in Limb Trauma Management

Splinting plays a crucial role throughout the care of limb trauma, from the scene of injury to long-term rehabilitation. Its primary functions include enhancing communication, providing pain relief, controlling hemorrhage, protecting tissues, immobilizing the affected area, aiding in transport, and potentially reducing the risk of fat embolism. In cases of limb trauma, splinted areas should be assumed to be fractured until proven otherwise. Splints should be documented and removed when appropriate to allow for a comprehensive assessment of the entire limb.

Pain relief is achieved through reducing movement in injured tissues. Proper splinting helps to minimize bleeding and edema, as well as ensure optimal bone alignment, which further reduces the risk of fracture-related bleeding. Additionally, splints protect injured tissues during transportation, allowing for safer movement to definitive care. While the role of early splinting in reducing fat embolism is debated, it remains a consideration in the initial trauma response.

Splints can be categorized based on location or type. For instance, general splints like spine boards or localized splints such as cervical collars are used to immobilize affected areas.

Splints may also be classified as anatomical (using the unaffected limb), soft, rigid, air, or sling-based splints. Despite their benefits, splints can introduce complications, such as skin pressure sores, compartment syndrome, loss of limb function, or impaired distal circulation. Therefore, splints should be removed for thorough inspection and reassessment of the limb.

Definitive fracture and dislocation management includes reduction, immobilization, and rehabilitation. Early reduction is beneficial in reducing pain by relieving pressure on nearby tissues and nerves. Furthermore, it helps avoid skin pressure and neurovascular damage. Deformities in limbs with compressed skin should be corrected as an orthopedic emergency, before imaging. For suspected joint injuries, definitive exploration should occur under general anesthesia.

In pre-hospital care, injured limbs should be immobilized in a neutral or anatomical position, whenever possible, with joints above and below the injury also secured. Specific injuries like femoral shaft fractures may require traction to counteract muscle spasms. Devices such as the CT-6 or Kendrick traction device can be employed. After splinting, the distal neurovascular status of the limb should be reassessed.

Rehabilitation starts in the emergency department (ED), where early movement of uninjured limbs is encouraged. The use of crutches and the care of slings can help patients regain mobility and reduce complications. Follow-up care is essential for monitoring fractures and other high-risk injuries. Discharge from the ED occurs when limb and life-threatening injuries have been excluded, and the patient is ambulatory, tolerating food, and has follow-up arrangements.

Wound Management

The effectiveness of wound irrigation agents in acute trauma remains contentious. Full-strength povidone-iodine should be avoided, as it delays healing and increases infection risks. If used, it should be diluted to less than 1%. Shaving of wounds is discouraged due to its potential to cause local inflammation. Instead, normal saline should be used for irrigation, with the pressure of 7 to 10 psi (48 to 69 kPa) to effectively remove debris and bacteria without spreading microorganisms. High-pressure irrigation does not offer additional benefits.

Managing the Mangled Extremity

The mangled extremity requires prompt attention, focusing on life-threatening injuries while simultaneously addressing the limb's anatomical alignment and vascular and nerve health. The goals of management include controlling bleeding with direct pressure or, if unsuccessful, using a tourniquet as a temporary measure. Timely reperfusion of ischemic tissues, early reduction of long bone fractures, and adequate analgesia are crucial steps. Repeated doses of fentanyl or ketamine are commonly used to manage pain during manipulation of fractures. Communication with surgical specialists is essential for timely operative intervention.

Hyperbaric Oxygen Therapy (HBOT)

The use of HBOT for acute limb injuries remains debated. It is thought to enhance oxygen delivery to hypoxic tissues affected by edema, potentially reducing the extent of ischemia and necrosis. Some studies show benefit in managing crush injuries, compartment syndrome, and non-union fractures. Though indications for HBOT are listed by the US Hyperbaric Society, its practice varies by region.

Disposition and Post-Trauma Care

The ED is a critical care environment where patients are either discharged, admitted to a general ward, or transferred to surgery or the ICU. Following stabilization, patients may require further diagnostic imaging or transfer for procedures like angiography or

CT scans. For those discharged, a clear care plan should be provided, and follow-up arranged with relevant specialists. Elderly patients with splints should be assessed for mobilization safety, with the allied health team providing necessary aids. Oral analgesics should be prescribed for at least a week, with special attention given to covering weekends and holidays. Non-steroidal anti-inflammatory drugs (NSAIDs) should be avoided in older patients, as they can cause harm and provide no added benefit.

Patients with plaster casts should have documented evaluations of the cast, splints, and mobility aids, such as crutches. Upper limb slings should have cushioned supports to avoid pressure on the neck. Injured limbs should be elevated for the first 48 hours, with specific instructions for leg elevation when sitting or lying down. Patients should be instructed to return if their injury worsens or if there are signs of circulation issues, such as numbness, pallor, or increased pain.

Surgical Intervention and Operating Theatre Procedures

Urgent surgical intervention is required in cases of uncontrollable hemorrhage, severely contaminated wounds or open fractures, ischemic limbs lasting over 6 to 8 hours, crushed limbs requiring amputation, or infected limbs that may require amputation to save life. In patients with complex injuries or those at high surgical risk, damage-control surgery may be necessary. This approach involves temporarily stabilizing fractures and preparing the patient for a secondary procedure once their overall condition has improved. The goal of damage-control surgery is to manage hemorrhage, contamination, and swelling, reducing the risk of skin necrosis and fat embolism syndrome (FES).

Complications

Compartment Syndrome

Acute limb compartment syndrome (ALCS) is a serious

complication of trauma, caused by bleeding or edema within a closed muscle compartment. If untreated, it can result in muscle necrosis, limb loss, and potentially life-threatening complications, such as acute renal failure. Clinical signs include severe, disproportionate pain that worsens with passive movement of the injured limb, as well as firm, tense muscle compartments. Early recognition and treatment, including fasciotomy, are essential to prevent irreversible damage. Monitoring compartment pressures and relieving any restrictive splints are important interventions.

Common sites for compartment syndrome include the leg, thigh, and forearm, though it can also affect other areas like the buttocks and hands. The threshold for fasciotomy remains a point of debate, but most centers agree that intervention is required when compartment pressure exceeds 30 mmHg or if ischemia persists.

Immobilization

Certain patients may need extended periods of immobilization, which can occur in a hospital setting, rehabilitation centers, or at home. The effects of prolonged immobility can include the development of pressure sores and skin damage, muscle wasting and weakness (which may increase the risk of falls), postural hypotension, atelectasis, and secondary pneumonia. Additional complications can include constipation, sleep disturbances, social isolation, and depression. A comprehensive management plan, which is clearly communicated and documented, can help prevent and address many of these issues.

Radiation Hazards in Trauma Care

The trauma team must adopt measures to limit unnecessary exposure to ionizing radiation. Ensuring that patients receive the least amount of radiation required for accurate diagnosis is crucial, adhering to the "As

Low As Reasonably Achievable" (ALARA) principle. Radiographic examinations, such as X-rays, should be minimized in the resuscitation setting to avoid excessive exposure. Since radiation exposure decreases with the square of the distance from the source, staff should position themselves at the greatest possible distance from the X-ray equipment when it is in use. In addition, using permanent lead barriers can further reduce exposure.

Ionizing radiation, which is used in X-rays and computed tomography (CT) scans, has the potential to directly or indirectly damage DNA. This damage may evade the body's natural repair mechanisms, contributing to an elevated risk of cancer. A 20-year study in Australia (1985-2005) demonstrated that patients who were exposed to ionizing radiation from CT scans had a 24% higher incidence of cancer compared to those not exposed, with the risk being more significant for those who were younger at the time of exposure. The increased cancer risk spanned multiple solid organ cancers and blood cancers. Based on these findings, the researchers recommended limiting CT scans to instances with clear clinical indications, ensuring that each scan is optimized to deliver the lowest possible radiation dose while achieving the necessary diagnostic quality.

The amount of radiation patients receive from various diagnostic imaging procedures can be quantified using an "effective dose," measured in millisieverts (mSv). This measure averages the radiation dose across the body, taking into account the varying sensitivities of different tissues. For instance, a single CT scan can deliver a dose between 10 and 30 mSv. The US Food and Drug Administration estimates that a CT scan with an effective dose of 10 mSv carries a 1 in 2,000 lifetime risk of causing fatal cancer.

Trauma Imaging Protocols

In trauma care, the initial imaging typically includes a supine chest X-ray and pelvic X-ray. A lateral cervical spine X-ray may offer limited diagnostic value, while a CT scan of the cervical spine (from occiput to T4–T5) with sagittal and coronal reconstructions is necessary to comprehensively evaluate potential bony injuries. The CT scan should include the occipital condyles and the atlanto-axial junction to ensure thorough assessment.

Chest X-rays are usually performed in the supine antero-posterior (AP) position rather than the erect postero-anterior (PA) position because patients often cannot sit up until their spine has been cleared. A well-penetrated X-ray should capture both clavicles, the ribs, lungs, mediastinum, and diaphragm. When properly executed, a chest X-ray can identify serious injuries such as massive hemothorax, pneumothorax, multiple rib fractures, or a widened mediastinum.

Key Points for Trauma Imaging:

1. Initial trauma imaging should include a chest X-ray (CXR) and pelvic X-ray (PXR). CT scans of the cervical spine are essential to rule out fractures or dislocations.

2. CT of the brain is crucial for detecting most types of intracranial hemorrhage, but diffuse axonal injury (DAI) is best identified through magnetic resonance imaging (MRI).

3. A CT scan of the cervical spine is critical for detecting bony injuries but will not reveal ligamentous, disc, or spinal cord damage.

4. If ligamentous, disc, or spinal cord injuries are suspected, MRI is necessary.

5. A CT of the facial bones is essential to rule out bony injuries in the facial region.

6. Unconscious trauma patients may require a whole-body CT scan to evaluate injuries that are difficult to assess through physical examination alone. Clinical judgment should always precede such imaging decisions.

7. Conscious trauma patients should only undergo CT scans of areas that show clinical signs of injury.

8. CT scans are typically sufficient to rule out chest, abdominal, or pelvic injuries, with or without the use of intravenous contrast.

9. Injuries to the thoracolumbar spine should be assessed with sagittal and coronal reconstructions of axial CT scans from the chest, abdomen, or pelvis.

10. A CT angiogram is the preferred imaging modality if blunt cerebrovascular injury (BCVI) is suspected based on relevant clinical indicators.

11. The clinical team must balance the risks of radiation exposure for both the patient and medical staff, especially when considering CT scans for pediatric patients.

Head Trauma Imaging

Head trauma is responsible for a significant proportion of pre-hospital trauma-related fatalities, with varying degrees of severity. Mild concussions, moderate brain injuries, and severe trauma, such as diffuse axonal injury (DAI), all fall within the spectrum of head injuries, including various types of intracranial hemorrhage.

For most significant head injuries, a CT scan of the brain is the preferred imaging modality, as it can detect intracranial hematomas, cerebral edema (with or without midline shift), and skull fractures. The Canadian CT Head Rule guides CT scanning decisions in cases of minor head injury, using high- and medium-risk factors to determine the need for neurological intervention. For example, the presence of specific high-risk factors ensures a 100% sensitivity for predicting the need for further intervention, while medium-risk factors detect clinically important brain injuries with a 97.2% sensitivity.

MRI is considered the gold standard for diagnosing DAI, as it offers superior sensitivity for detecting contusions, shear injuries, and extra-axial hematomas compared to CT.

MRI is particularly effective in identifying white matter lesions caused by shear injuries, which may not be visible on CT scans.

Classification of Intracranial Hemorrhage

Intracranial hemorrhage can be classified by location, such as subdural, subarachnoid, extradural, intraventricular, or parenchymal bleeding. These types of hemorrhage often occur together in trauma cases.

Extradural Hematomas: Typically result from arterial bleeding due to skull fractures that disrupt the middle meningeal artery. The hematoma appears as an ovoid or lentiform shape and does not cross cranial sutures but may cross the midline.

Subdural Hematomas: Usually result from venous bleeding and appear crescentic. These may extend across sutures but not the midline.

Subarachnoid Hemorrhage: Often caused by the rupture of small vessels or extension from a parenchymal contusion/hematoma. It appears in the sulci or cisterns around the brain.

Intraventricular Hemorrhage: Results from the rupture of subependymal veins or extension from parenchymal hemorrhage, with blood products layering in dependent areas on CT scans.

Cerebral Contusions: Represent localized brain bleeds and often increase in size and number in the first 24 hours following trauma.

Additionally, head injuries in patients on anticoagulants or antiplatelet therapy may result in progressively worsening hemorrhages over the first 24 hours, which can occur in multiple locations despite attempts at pharmacological or surgical intervention.

Emergency Department (ED) Wound Management: A Comprehensive Overview

Unintentional injuries, including cutting and piercing wounds, are a significant component of the emergency department (ED) workload. Data from the Victorian Injury Surveillance System reveals that 72% of ED visits for these injuries do not require hospital admission and typically involve open wounds. Furthermore, open wounds may coexist with other injuries, such as fractures. Specifically, 19% of home-related open wounds occur in the pediatric age group (0–14 years), 62% in individuals under 35 years, and fewer than 10% in those over 65. Notably, 65% of the affected patients are male. Geographically, over 53% of these injuries occur in the home, primarily during leisure activities. The leading causes include falls (under 1 meter), contact with sharp objects, and collisions. The majority of these injuries are unintentional, with only 3% attributed to assault. Facial, head, and neck injuries account for 12% of the cases, while upper extremity injuries are most common, comprising 62%. About 88% of these wounds are treated and repaired in the ED, with many patients subsequently discharged, while nearly half are referred to general practitioners or specialists for follow-up care.

Clinical Assessment and Wound Management

A thorough initial assessment is critical in determining the appropriate treatment approach for open wounds. This assessment involves a detailed history, physical examination, and investigation to evaluate the wound and surrounding areas for potential complications. Key aspects of the history include the mechanism of injury, the time of occurrence, possible foreign body presence, and the patient's immunization status (especially tetanus). Past medical history, allergies to certain medications, and current medications such as anticoagulants or cytotoxic drugs should also be noted, as these factors influence the management and healing process.

For example, diabetic patients are at a higher risk of infection and poor wound healing, especially in extremity injuries. In addition, conditions such as prior mastectomy, splenectomy, liver dysfunction, immunosuppressive treatments, or autoimmune diseases (e.g., systemic lupus erythematosus) may increase the risk of complications, particularly in contaminated wounds like bites. Smokers, due to impaired collagen production, also face challenges in wound healing.

The physical examination must include an overall assessment for other injuries and concurrent medical conditions, such as poor circulation in patients with peripheral vascular disease. The area surrounding the wound should be thoroughly examined to check for constricting rings or jewelry, which should be removed to ensure unhindered examination. After a general assessment, a local examination of the wound is necessary, followed by cleaning to remove contaminants. Evaluation for nerve or vascular damage should be conducted, and if needed, further imaging (e.g., radiographs or ultrasound) may be ordered to check for foreign bodies or fractures.

Wound Cleaning and Repair

Proper wound cleaning is crucial for optimal healing and to prevent infection. This involves removing all contaminants, foreign bodies, and necrotic tissue before closing the wound. Several key principles guide wound repair:

1. Cosmetic Outcomes: Good cosmetic outcomes can often be achieved through conservative treatment, meticulous debridement, and precise approximation of the wound edges.

2. Suture Selection: Monofilament sutures, which cause minimal tissue reaction and maintain tensile strength until the wound heals, are preferred.

3. Timeliness: In contaminated wounds, it is important to cleanse, debride, and close the wound within 6 hours to minimize infection risk.

4. Tendon Injuries: Suspected tendon injuries should be evaluated by assessing the full range of motion in the affected joint. Any damage to tendons or nerves should prompt

referral to a specialist, such as a plastic surgeon.

5. Postoperative Care: Effective postoperative care, including physical therapy and splinting, is crucial for tendon repair success.

6. Antibiotics and Infection Control: The use of antibiotics is recommended in cases involving joint, tendon, nerve, or significant crush injuries, as well as bites. However, simple lacerations without these complications generally do not require antibiotics.

For wounds involving body cavities (e.g., peritoneum, joints) or critical structures (e.g., flexor tendons, major arteries), referral to a specialist is necessary. Similarly, puncture wounds and those with embedded foreign bodies may require special care, including excisional debridement and targeted closure techniques.

Wound Cleaning Procedures

Before cleaning, the area should be protected with appropriate personal protective equipment (PPE), including gloves, gowns, and eye protection. Gloves should be powder-free to prevent the introduction of starch, which could complicate wound healing. Hair may be clipped, not shaved, as shaving can damage hair follicles and increase infection risk. Sterile saline is the preferred cleansing solution due to its low toxicity, although recent studies suggest that tap water is equally effective for simple lacerations. For more contaminated or extensive wounds, local anesthesia is necessary. In cases of heavy contamination, such as with road debris, general anesthesia may be required. Wounds should be irrigated with pressure of at least 8 psi to dislodge bacteria and reduce infection risk. Foreign bodies, such as gravel or metal, can be detected with radiographs, while ultrasound may help identify non-radiopaque materials like wood, provided they are larger than 2.5 mm. Debridement should be performed carefully, with emphasis on removing only necrotic tissue and preserving healthy tissue. The approach has shifted from aggressive to more selective debridement, which helps minimize damage to viable tissues. For instance, muscle, nerves, and major vessels should not be aggressively debrided in the ED.

Tetanus Prophylaxis and Wound Healing

Tetanus remains a serious concern, especially in older adults who may have neglected their immunizations. Clostridium tetani, a bacterium found in soil and animal feces, produces toxins that lead to severe muscle spasms and potentially fatal respiratory failure. Tetanus immunoglobulin should be administered to patients with inadequate tetanus protection, in addition to tetanus toxoid for active immunity.

Wound healing proceeds through three phases:

Lag Phase (Days 1-5): No significant strength gain occurs during this period, and inflammation is predominant.

Proliferative Phase (Days 5-14): The wound strength increases rapidly due to fibroplasia and epithelialization.

Maturation Phase (Post-Day 14): Collagen remodeling continues, with the wound never regaining more than 80% of the original skin strength.

Secondary healing (healing by second intention) may occur when wounds are left to heal naturally, particularly in the case of contamination or tension. However, consultation with a plastic surgeon is recommended when there is uncertainty about the appropriate method of wound closure.

In conclusion, the management of open wounds in the ED requires a systematic and thorough approach to ensure optimal healing outcomes. Wound assessment, cleaning, debridement, and timely closure, along with appropriate use of antibiotics, tetanus prophylaxis, and postoperative care, are all critical to minimizing complications and promoting effective recovery.

Needle and Suture Selection

For denser tissues such as tendons or aponeuroses, needles with a combination of a cutting point at the tip and a taper for the body are recommended. Needle holders are typically used with curved needles, while straight needles are generally held by hand. The use of straight, handheld needles carries the risk of needle-stick injuries, making them potentially hazardous.

Basic Suture Technique

Before starting the closure, intravenous prophylactic antibiotics (refer to Chapter 9.9) should be administered as needed to reduce the risk of infection, especially if a hematoma forms during or after closure. Once a sterile field is prepared, the suture tray (Box 3.10.3) is set up, and the wound is anesthetized, cleaned, and draped, the repair process can begin. For a heavily contaminated wound, anesthesia, lavage, and debridement are essential before antiseptic preparation and draping for formal closure.

The suture selected should be as thin as possible while still providing the necessary strength to withstand tissue tension. The needle holder should grasp the needle about two-thirds of the way from its tip, avoiding the weaker swage. To make handling easier, stretching the suture and supporting it at the needle swage can eliminate its "memory." The needle holder is held in the palm and controlled with the index finger, using a supination/pronation motion to guide the needle along its arc.

For small linear wounds, a straightforward approach of suturing from one end to the other may suffice. In longer wounds lacking clear landmarks, dividing the wound into sections ensures even closure and prevents a "dog-ear" formation. Stretching the wound with the help of an assistant can aid in achieving an even closure. In more complex or irregular wounds, it's helpful to begin by approximating corresponding landmarks, such as stitching the apex of a flap first.

After wound contraction, the skin tends to invert, creating a shallow crater. To avoid this, the edges must be everted at closure, either by pressing on the skin near the wound edge or lifting it with a skin hook or forceps. The needle should enter and exit perpendicularly to the skin for both running and interrupted sutures. Sutures can be placed as interrupted or continuous loops, with vertical mattress sutures used for edges difficult to maintain inversion with simple sutures.

Knot Techniques

Knots are typically the weakest part of a suture, particularly in continuous sutures, where knot failure can cause the entire suture to fail along the wound. When tying knots, care must be taken not to damage the suture by crushing it with the serrated jaws of a needle holder. A reef knot with a snug third throw provides the best results for materials like nylon or polypropylene. Synthetic monofilament sutures require several twists in the first two throws to prevent untying.

It's critical that sutures are not tied too tightly, as this can lead to ischaemia and cause skin surface marks. To avoid strangulation of tissue, one method is to use a loop throw in interrupted sutures. Studies indicate no significant increase in infection or decrease in wound strength when using continuous sutures, which distribute tension evenly and are quicker to place. However, if a single knot fails, the whole suture line can loosen. Intradermal sutures are particularly useful for surgical wounds and should be spaced about 3 cm apart to facilitate removal.

Suture Removal and Handling
Monofilament absorbable sutures, like glycolide caprolactone (Monocryl), have replaced polypropylene for continuous subcuticular closures due to their easier handling and the fact that they don't require removal. It is important to ensure the suture

glides smoothly during placement and isn't looped, as this can make removal challenging.

Closing Wounds and Managing Dead Space

Historically, it was emphasized to eliminate dead space within a wound to prevent infection. However, more recent studies have shown that suture closure of dead space may actually increase infection risk, as the suture acts as a foreign body in the wound. Therefore, it's now preferred to leave some dead space open to avoid complications.

Buried sutures are sometimes used to promote wound-edge eversion and close deep spaces. Modern sutures allow for this without leaving a risk of infection. Proper dermal edge apposition, whether using deep sutures or not, remains key to achieving the narrowest possible scar.

Special Considerations in Suture Techniques

In cases where the wound involves thick skin, such as on the back, trimming the edges with a scalpel perpendicular to the skin or using vertical mattress sutures can prevent one beveled edge from sliding over another. Adjustments to the height of the wound edges can be made using the needle to exit more superficially on the high side and deeper on the low side.

Specialized Wound Closure

In scalp lacerations, the "hair braiding" technique can be effective. This involves twisting several strands of hair from opposite sides and securing them with tissue adhesive. For facial wounds, early closure is essential for optimal cosmetic results, and in some cases, the wound can be temporarily cleaned and dressed until definitive repair can be performed.

In ear injuries, alignment of cartilage and skin coverage is vital to prevent perichondritis. Eyelid injuries require careful examination to rule out scleral or conjunctival damage and should involve immediate micro-surgical repair if canaliculi are affected. Special care is needed for facial injuries, with attention to facial symmetry and checking for facial nerve and parotid duct integrity.

Special Suture Techniques for Tension Relief

For wounds with high tension, techniques like limited undermining and horizontal mattress sutures can be useful. Skin flaps are rarely raised in acute trauma but may be used in certain situations to relieve tension. However, split skin grafts are often preferred for wound healing, with subsequent scar revision performed later.

Managing "Dog-Ears"

A "dog-ear" refers to a conical pucker of redundant skin that forms at the end of a wound, particularly in elliptical skin defects. To avoid this, the wound should be sutured in halves, with each new stitch placed between the previous ones. If a dog-ear forms, it can be removed using techniques such as direct overlap excision or V-Y excision, depending on the size and location of the redundancy.

Drainage

Wound drainage is necessary to prevent infection, fluid accumulation, and pressure on surrounding vasculature. There are two main types of drains: active suction drains and passive drains. Suction drains are generally more effective, but they may become blocked. A simple suction drain can be constructed from a "butterfly" cannula and a vacuum blood specimen tube, ensuring fluid removal while maintaining a sterile environment.

Chapter 8 (G)
Burns

Introduction

In recent decades, advancements in burn care have greatly lowered mortality rates and enhanced the quality of life for burn survivors. Effective strategies such as timely fluid resuscitation, early wound debridement, and the prudent application of antibiotics have mitigated common burn-related complications like hypovolemia and sepsis. However, mortality in burn cases now often stems from multi-organ failure, with significant risk factors including patient age, total burn surface area, inhalation injuries, and female gender.

Pathophysiology

The skin, as the body's largest organ, plays crucial roles including serving as a barrier to prevent fluid loss, protect against infections, and regulate temperature. Structurally, it comprises two main layers: the epidermis, which is vital for minimizing passive water loss, and the dermis, housing sweat glands, hair follicles, sebaceous glands, sensory receptors, and blood vessels, which collectively aid in thermoregulation. Burn injuries can lead to coagulative necrosis of the skin, resulting in distinct zones: a central zone of irreversible cell damage, a surrounding zone of stasis prone to ischemia, and an outer hyperemic zone. Early, targeted intervention can limit damage progression.

Classification of Burns

Burns are classified by depth into epidermal, partial-thickness (subdivided into superficial, mid-dermal, and deep), and full-thickness categories. Superficial burns, affecting only the epidermis, tend to heal within a week. Partial-thickness burns, which affect both the epidermis and dermis, vary in severity. Superficial partial-thickness burns are bright red, sensitive, and typically heal within 2–3 weeks, while deep partial-thickness burns, often dark red or yellowish, take longer to heal and are prone to scarring. Full-thickness burns extend through both skin layers and require grafting or scar tissue formation for healing.

Thermal Burns: Presentation and Initial Evaluation

In assessing burn injuries, a thorough history—including details of the burn's cause, exposure duration, and any involvement of enclosed spaces—is critical. Symptoms like altered consciousness, confinement to a burning environment, and presence of inhaled smoke suggest carbon monoxide poisoning. During examination, signs such as facial burns, singed nasal hair, or carbonaceous sputum point to inhalation injuries. Immediate assessment should also consider possible airway obstruction due to laryngeal edema, as well as circumferential limb burns that may compromise circulation.

Evaluation of Burn Area

Accurate assessment of burn size and depth is essential for proper management. The "rule of nines" is commonly used for adults, while the Lund and Browder chart provides adjustments for infants and children. The palm method, where the patient's palm represents 1% of body surface area, is suitable for estimating smaller burns.

Management

Pre-Hospital Care

Pre-hospital management should focus on extinguishing the burn source, stabilizing the airway, breathing, and circulation, and quickly transporting the patient to a burn center if necessary. Application of cool running water for 20 minutes is recommended for partial-thickness burns, but direct ice application should be avoided to prevent deepening the burn. Ensuring warmth and administering supplemental oxygen are critical, and if transport is prolonged, intravenous fluids may be needed.

Emergency Department Care

In the emergency setting, oxygen therapy and continuous monitoring are priorities. Securing the airway and managing life-threatening injuries precede wound care. Burns involving the face, neck, or airway require prompt intubation to prevent edema-related airway obstruction. For burn patients with suspected inhalation injury, bronchodilators may be required to alleviate bronchospasm induced by smoke particles. Carbon monoxide poisoning should be suspected with symptoms such as tachypnea, confusion, and cherry-red mucous membranes; high-flow oxygen can reduce CO dissociation time, aiding recovery.

Fluid Resuscitation

Intravenous fluid administration is essential for stabilizing burn patients, especially those with extensive injuries. Fluid resuscitation protocols, using crystalloid solutions, help maintain circulatory stability and prevent further organ damage.

Subsequent Management of Burn Patients

Once a burn patient is stabilized and fluid resuscitation is initiated, a comprehensive secondary survey should assess any additional injuries. Pain management is a critical component; smaller burns may be treated with cool compresses and oral analgesics, while extensive burns may require parenteral analgesics, often utilizing opiates. For persistent pain control, a ketamine infusion may be advantageous, especially for severe burns.

Burn victims are prone to rapid heat loss, necessitating

measures such as wrapping in blankets, foil, or warming devices to prevent hypothermia. Initial wound care can be achieved with cling film, which serves as a protective, non-adherent barrier, providing pain relief and allowing visual assessment of burn severity. Deep burns and eschars often benefit from early surgical interventions like excision and autologous skin grafting. Tangential escharotomy, which selectively removes necrotic tissue while preserving healthy tissue, is commonly applied to deep burns. Circumferential burns, particularly on the limbs, may necessitate escharotomy to prevent ischemic necrosis when pulses are absent. For circumferential chest burns, escharotomy can also be essential to alleviate chest wall restriction and support ventilation.

For patients with facial burns, fluorescein staining is recommended to facilitate early diagnosis and treatment of potential corneal damage. Additionally, tetanus prophylaxis should be administered to those without a booster in the past decade, with tetanus immunoglobulin for wounds heavily contaminated with soil. Routine systemic antibiotics are not indicated, although selective use may be considered for immunocompromised patients.

Burn Shock and Pathophysiology

Burn shock is characterized by complex pathophysiological changes, including fluid shifts, coagulopathy, and cardiac output reduction. Within the first 8 hours post-burn, inflammatory mediators like prostaglandins and leukotrienes increase capillary permeability, leading to significant tissue edema. Burned tissues undergo osmotically driven fluid shifts due to cellular breakdown and collagen degradation, exacerbating edema. The combination of tissue injury and fluid dilution contributes to coagulation dysfunction, which affects approximately one-third of severe burn patients. Additionally, the loss of skin integrity results in substantial evaporative fluid loss, while cardiac output can decrease by 30-50% in major burns, potentially due to circulating myocardial depressant factors.

Inhalation Injury

Inhalation injuries significantly worsen burn outcomes, typically resulting from inhaling toxic combustion products rather than direct thermal damage. Common complications arise from smoke exposure, which contains particulates (mainly carbon) and various gasses like carbon monoxide, hydrogen cyanide, and oxides of nitrogen and sulfur. These compounds adhere to respiratory mucosa, causing irritation, hypersecretion, and potential airway obstruction. The inhaled toxins can also lead to increased pulmonary artery pressures due to thromboxane release, contributing to respiratory complications.

Disposition and Transfer Guidelines

Patients with severe burns should ideally be treated in

specialized burn units. Coordination with the receiving unit ensures that the patient receives appropriate stabilization prior to transfer. For transport, applying cling film over burns reduces heat and fluid loss without impeding later evaluations. Silver sulfadiazine (SSD) cream should be avoided on major burns as it may interfere with subsequent assessments.

Current burn management for deep partial-thickness and full-thickness burns often involves prompt excision and grafting. In cases of extensive burns, grafting may be done in stages to allow for skin regeneration. Minor burns can be managed with various dressing options, including alginate, foam, and hydrocolloid dressings, which support moist wound healing and reduce trauma during dressing changes. Outpatient management may be appropriate for superficial burns covering less than 10% of total body surface area (TBSA), provided patients meet specific social and psychological criteria.

Management of Chemical Burns

Chemical burns can range from superficial irritation to deep tissue destruction, depending on the chemical's nature, concentration, and exposure duration. Acids typically cause coagulation necrosis, limiting tissue damage, while alkalis induce liquefactive necrosis, leading to deeper penetration. Treatment begins with decontamination—removing contaminated clothing and thoroughly irrigating the affected area. For alkali burns, extended irrigation is often necessary to neutralize tissue penetration. Litmus paper can help guide irrigation duration by indicating wound pH.

Disposition Criteria for Chemical Burns

Most chemical burn cases are manageable on an outpatient basis. However, hospitalization is required for:

Partial-thickness burns covering >15% TBSA

Any full-thickness burns

Burns involving critical areas (hands, feet, face, perineum)

Cases with systemic toxicity or significant comorbidities

Massive Transfusion: An Overview and Clinical Approach

A massive transfusion (MT) typically refers to the rapid replacement of a significant volume of a patient's blood. For a standard adult weighing approximately 70 kg, the average blood volume is around 5 liters, with a red cell volume ranging between 2 to 2.5 liters, assuming a hematocrit of 0.40-0.50. In clinical terms, MT is traditionally defined as administering at least 10 units of packed red blood cells (PRBCs) within 24 hours—an estimation based on total red cell volume requirements for a 70-kg adult.

However, recent research suggests that this definition may not accurately reflect the needs of acutely bleeding patients. Patients at risk of death before reaching the 10-unit threshold are often overlooked, as are those who might require rapid transfusion within shorter time frames, such as at least 5 units in 4 hours or over 10 units in 6 hours. These alternative criteria have been introduced to better identify patients requiring aggressive and immediate intervention.

Guidelines for MT Activation

In clinical practice, early identification of MT candidates and timely activation of MT protocols are essential. Effective systems for MT prenotification should be established, especially for patients arriving with high hemorrhage risk. An interdisciplinary team approach is critical, with the emergency physician generally serving as team leader. Given that laboratory test results may be delayed and are often unreliable during conditions of acidosis or hypothermia, MT protocols must be proactive and evidence-informed.

Challenges in Transfusion Practices

Patients undergoing MT often face increased mortality risks, especially those with coagulopathy, who are four times more likely to die compared to those without. Transfusions are linked to various complications, such as acute respiratory distress syndrome (ARDS), multi-organ failure, minor allergic reactions, and infections. To mitigate these risks and manage limited blood resources, modern resuscitation strategies emphasize restrictive transfusion practices, hemorrhage control, and correction of coagulopathies through precise blood product ratios and goal-directed management.

Prediction and Preparation for MT

Predicting the need for MT, especially in trauma settings, has led to the development of several scoring tools. These scores, though high in specificity, often have limited sensitivity. Thus, MT protocols should be activated based on clinical judgment rather than solely relying on predictive scores. Preparatory measures for MT involve prompt communication from prehospital providers, notification of relevant staff, and allocation of roles under the team leader's direction.

Patient Reception and Monitoring

Upon arrival, patients requiring MT should be assessed in designated trauma or resuscitation units with comprehensive physiological monitoring. Immediate diagnostic and management steps, such as focused assessment with sonography for trauma (FAST) in hemodynamically unstable cases, should be conducted by credentialed personnel.

Essential History and Investigations

Key historical factors include the patient's age, mechanism of injury, and bleeding history, as well as prior transfusion reactions or coagulopathies. Laboratory tests, although sometimes delayed, should include blood grouping, cross-matching, full blood counts, and coagulation studies. Near-patient tests, like thromboelastography (TEG) and rotational thromboelastometry (ROTEM), offer rapid insights into coagulopathy and can be particularly useful in MT management.

Massive Transfusion Guidelines

A clinical guideline is a structured statement that aids healthcare providers in making informed decisions regarding specific patient scenarios. Due to diverse evidence levels surrounding the management of massive hemorrhage, transfusion guidelines vary widely across regions. However, certain core elements are commonly upheld.

Fresh Frozen Plasma (FFP)

FFP is integral to massive transfusion (MT) protocols, particularly supported by trauma resuscitation data. A pivotal study by Borgman et al. in 2006 examined combat casualties in Baghdad who received 10 or more units of packed red blood cells (PRBCs) or whole blood within 24 hours.

Patients were stratified by low (1:12–1:5), intermediate (1:3.0–1:2.3), and high (1:1.7–1:1.2) FFP:PRBC ratios, showing an overall mortality of 28%. However, the mortality in the high FFP ratio group was significantly lower at 19%. While this study had limitations, including its retrospective design and the use of whole blood in a military setting, it underscored a potentially life-saving approach through high-ratio plasma use.

Subsequent retrospective studies have explored high FFP:PRBC ratios in trauma care, though survival bias and inadequate controls limit their conclusions. Observational data suggests that those surviving severe trauma may simply receive more FFP, rather than high FFP:PRBC ratios actively contributing to survival. Current recommendations advise early FFP administration in massive hemorrhage cases at a dose of 10-15 mL/kg, with adjustments based on coagulation monitoring and additional blood product requirements. Evidence supports a minimum FFP:PRBC ratio of 1:2 when ongoing PRBC transfusions are needed.

Platelet Transfusion

The early use of platelets in hemorrhagic shock management remains debated. Platelets are collected through apheresis, which isolates platelets and plasma from whole blood, or from pooled whole blood from multiple donors. In Australia, both apheresis and pooled platelets are typically irradiated before release.

Historical studies suggested that a platelet count of $100,000/mm^3$ marks the threshold for significant bleeding. In contrast, recent guidelines maintain that a minimum threshold of $50,000/mm^3$ is often adequate, although patients with severe trauma or massive hemorrhage may benefit from a target of $100,000/mm^3$. Platelet functionality, beyond just count, is critical, as coagulation relies on thrombin activity to sustain clot stability. Evidence remains insufficient for a specific platelet transfusion threshold, suggesting that decisions be made with a low threshold for transfusion without rigid cut-offs.

Cryoprecipitate

Evidence supporting cryoprecipitate use during MT is limited, though it effectively increases fibrinogen and von Willebrand factor concentrations. Administration is recommended when fibrinogen levels fall below 1.0 g/L, yet the clinical impact of maintaining higher-than-normal fibrinogen levels is still under investigation.

Calcium

Ionized calcium, a critical cofactor in coagulation, exists in both active (ionized) and inactive forms, with levels influenced by blood pH. Low ionized calcium can impair platelet function and cardiac contractility. During MT, hypocalcemia commonly results from citrate in blood products binding to ionized calcium, often observed in FFP and platelet transfusions. Monitoring ionized calcium levels is advised during MT, and calcium chloride should be administered if levels drop or hypocalcemic symptoms appear.

Synthetic Agents

Certain pharmacological agents can reduce bleeding by enhancing clot stability. Tranexamic acid (TXA), a synthetic antifibrinolytic, has demonstrated mortality reduction in trauma patients through the CRASH-2 trial, showing a 15% lower risk of death due to bleeding among TXA recipients. While TXA's benefit is established, its routine use in advanced trauma systems, where mortality rates are lower, is still debated. Prehospital trials are ongoing to assess TXA's effectiveness where acute traumatic coagulopathy (ATC) management is minimal. Recombinant activated factor VII (rFVIIa) is another agent with proven safety in surgical bleeding but is recommended only when standard measures fail.

Acute Traumatic Coagulopathy (ATC)

ATC, a distinct coagulopathy triggered by tissue damage and shock, is identified in nearly one-quarter of severe trauma cases. It is primarily measured by prolonged prothrombin time (PT), which reflects clotting factor function in the extrinsic pathway. Defining ATC and its relationship with trauma outcomes is vital for targeted resuscitation strategies in the severely injured.

References

1. Mitra B, Mori A, Cameron PA. Use of massive transfusion in trauma resuscitation. Injury. 2007;38(9):1023–1029.

2. Kashuk JL, Moore EE, Johnson JL. Life-threatening coagulopathy after trauma: can a 1:1 ratio of fresh frozen plasma to packed red blood cells improve outcomes? J Trauma. 2008;65:261–270.

3. Mitra B, Mori A, Cameron P. Application of fresh frozen plasma during trauma-related

massive transfusion. Injury. 2010;41:35–39.

4. Mitra B, Cameron PA, Gruen RL. The significance of defining massive transfusion in trauma research. Eur J Emerg Med. 2011;18:137–142.

5. Cotton BA, Au BK, Nunez TC. Impact of predefined massive transfusion protocols on reducing organ failure and trauma-related complications. J Trauma. 2009;66:41–48.

6. Cotton B, Dossett L, Au B. Analyzing provider factors influencing outcomes in massive transfusion procedures. J Trauma. 2009;67:1004–1012.

7. Marik PE, Corwin HL. Systematic review on red blood cell transfusion efficacy in critically ill patients. Crit Care Med. 2008;36:2667–2674.

8. Fitzgerald MC, Chan JY, Ross AW. Synthetic hemoglobin as a solution to cardiac hypoxia from severe anemia post-trauma. Med J Aust. 2011;194:471–473.

9. MacLeod JB, Lynn M, McKenney MG. Coagulopathy in early trauma as a predictor of

mortality. J Trauma. 2003;55:39–44.

10. Borgman MA, Spinella PC, Perkins JG. Effect of blood product ratios on mortality in massive transfusion at a combat support hospital. J Trauma. 2007;63:805–813.

11. Dutton RP, Mackenzie CF, Scalea TM. Hypotensive resuscitation in active hemorrhage: effects on hospital mortality. J Trauma. 2002;52:1141–1146.

12. Vivien B, Langeron O, Morell E. Hypocalcemia in severe trauma during initial treatment. Crit Care Med. 2005;33:1946–1952.

13. Mitra B, Cameron PA, Parr M, Phillips P. Use of recombinant factor VIIa in trauma patients with the "triad of death". Injury. 2012;43(9):1409–1414.

14. CRASH-2 trial collaborators. The impact of tranexamic acid on mortality, thrombotic events, and blood transfusion in severely bleeding trauma patients: results from the CRASH-2 trial. Lancet. 2010;376:23–32.

15. Gruen RL, Mitra B. Application of tranexamic acid in trauma cases. Lancet.

Chapter 9 (A)
Orthopedic Emergency

Clavicle Fractures

Clavicle fractures represent 2.6%-5% of all fractures, commonly caused by a direct shoulder impact or a fall on an outstretched arm. The middle third is the most frequently affected area (69%-82%). Displacement varies, and fractures often lead to fragment overlap and shortening. While injury to the pleura, axillary vessels, or brachial plexus is possible due to the clavicle's anatomical position, these are rare and should be ruled out through a targeted assessment.

Patients with clavicle fractures often support the injured arm at the elbow, with localized pain, tenderness, and sometimes visible deformity. Non-displaced or minimally displaced fractures typically require a sling for 2-3 weeks. Once pain subsides, early shoulder mobilization is encouraged, with immobilization ceasing upon clinical union, though radiological union may lag behind. Non-union is rare, but factors like complete displacement, comminution, and osteoporosis increase the risk, especially in elderly or osteoporotic women, who may benefit from surgical stabilization with plate-and-screw or intramedullary devices.

Outer clavicle fractures may involve the coracoclavicular ligaments and, if displaced, surgical intervention is advisable due to a high non-union rate (30%). Medial clavicle fractures are often associated with severe injuries, necessitating further investigation. Prompt orthopedic consultation is recommended for displaced fractures of the medial and outer clavicle regions. Late complications include stiffness and a localized lump, generally inconsequential cosmetically.

Key Points:

1. Most clavicular fractures heal without reduction.

2. Shoulder injuries may also impact neurovascular structures.

3. AC joint injuries and scapular fractures are usually managed conservatively.

4. Posterior sternoclavicular dislocations require reduction.

5. Shoulder dislocation requires axillary nerve and artery assessment.

6. Surgical repair is recommended for shoulder dislocation recurrences in active individuals.

Acromioclavicular Joint (AC) Injuries

AC joint injuries commonly result from falls onto the shoulder. The severity of the injury correlates with ligament damage and is categorized by the Tossy-Rockwood classification:

Type I: Partial tear of the AC ligament; CC ligament intact; no deformity.

Type II: Complete tear of the AC ligament; partial tear of the CC ligament; mild clavicle elevation.

Type III: Complete tear of both AC and CC ligaments; significant clavicle elevation.

Type IV-VI: Severe injury involving complete ligament and muscular attachments disruption.

AC dislocations are assessed clinically and by radiographic or ultrasonographic imaging. Minor injuries (Type I-II) require a sling for 1-2 weeks, avoiding strenuous activities to prevent progression to Type III. Management for Type III injuries is debated, while Types IV-VI typically require surgery.

Sternoclavicular Joint Dislocation

Sternoclavicular dislocations are rare and often stem from high-impact trauma. They may be anterior or posterior, with the latter risking damage to major vessels of the trachea. Anterior subluxations are often stable with conservative management. Posterior dislocations, however, require prompt intervention, typically closed reduction under anesthesia, and may need surgical stabilization if instability persists.

Scapular Fractures

Scapular fractures are uncommon (<1% of fractures) and usually indicate high-energy trauma, with 90% of cases presenting with other injuries. Blade fractures are often treated conservatively with a sling, though highly displaced fractures may require surgical intervention. Scapular neck fractures involving the glenoid may necessitate surgical repair. The "floating shoulder" injury pattern (scapular neck and clavicle fractures) presents a management challenge due to ambiguous surgical indications.

Supraspinatus Tendon Injuries

Supraspinatus tears, often occurring with age-related degeneration, are common and may follow minor trauma. Pain on abduction and weakness in external rotation, confirmed by the "empty can" test, suggests supraspinatus involvement. Non-operative management is generally preferred, but acute full-thickness tears may require surgery.

Shoulder Dislocation

Shoulder dislocation places the humeral head anterior, posterior, or inferior to the glenoid, with anterior dislocations being most common, typically from falls or sports injuries. Immediate evaluation of neurovascular integrity, particularly of the axillary nerve, is essential both pre- and post-reduction.

Young Patients and Surgery

For younger patients, surgery can be highly effective in lowering the risk of recurrent dislocation. While recurrence rates are low in elderly patients, younger patients experience recurrence in 64% to 68% of cases.

Reduction Techniques

Most anterior glenohumeral dislocations can be managed without anesthesia or procedural sedation, provided that adequate analgesia and a patient, careful technique are used. Intra-articular injection of lignocaine (lidocaine) is a safe and effective option as an alternative to sedation for shoulder reduction.

FARES Technique

This technique can be performed with the patient in either a supine or prone position. The provider holds the patient's wrist, applying traction to the affected limb while keeping it in a neutral position. Gentle, oscillating movements (5–10 cm) are applied anteriorly and posteriorly, with the limb gradually abducted. Once the limb reaches 90 degrees of abduction, it is externally rotated at the shoulder while continuing traction and oscillating movements. The reduction usually occurs at around 120 degrees of abduction, with an approximate success rate of 89%.

Spaso Technique

In the supine position, the affected arm is lifted vertically by holding the forearm or wrist, applying traction. The shoulder is externally rotated during this vertical traction, achieving reduction. If necessary, downward countertraction over the shoulder joint may be applied. This technique has a reported success rate of around 75%.

Modified Kocher Maneuver

With the arm held at the elbow to apply traction, the shoulder is gradually externally rotated, stopping if muscle spasm or resistance is encountered. External rotation to about 90 degrees is often achievable, and reduction typically occurs at this stage. The elbow is then adducted until it crosses the chest, followed by internal rotation until the hand reaches the opposite shoulder.

Scapular Manipulation

Traditionally performed with the patient in a prone position, this technique can also be done seated. The provider moves the scapula by medially displacing the inferior tip using thumb pressure while stabilizing the upper portion with the opposite hand.

Posterior Dislocation

Posterior shoulder dislocations are easily overlooked, particularly in unconscious patients. Causes include falls on an outstretched or internally rotated hand, frontal impact, seizures, and electrical injuries, with some cases presenting bilaterally. The dislocation may not be visible on standard AP radiographs, necessitating additional views. Reduction is achieved by applying traction in 90 degrees of abduction, followed by external rotation. Aftercare mirrors that of anterior dislocations.

Outcomes are generally favorable if the dislocation is detected and treated early, with a stable reduction and minimal bone damage. Poor prognostic indicators include delayed diagnosis, substantial humeral head defects, joint deformity, arthrosis, fractures near the proximal humerus, and the need for joint replacement. Surgical intervention remains a debated approach.

Inferior Dislocation (Luxatio Erecta)

This uncommon type of dislocation is often apparent due to the arm's abducted position. Neurovascular compromise is a significant concern, requiring thorough assessment and immediate reduction. Reduction is performed by traction in abduction, followed by movement into adduction. Post-reduction care follows the same guidelines as for anterior dislocation.

Chapter 9 (B)
Elbow Dislocations: A Detailed Analysis and Approach

Elbow dislocations rank among the top three most common large joint dislocations, alongside glenohumeral and patellofemoral joint dislocations, and are the second most frequent type of non-prosthetic joint dislocation. The elbow joint, a complex hinge structure, consists of the distal humerus, and the proximal radius and ulna. Given the strength of its surrounding muscles and ligaments, the elbow typically exhibits high stability, with most cases of dislocation resolvable without surgery, even if instability persists initially.

Classification of Elbow Dislocations

Elbow dislocations are primarily classified into anterior and posterior types:

1. Posterior Dislocations: The more prevalent type, often subdivided into postero-medial and postero-lateral categories. These frequently result from a fall on an outstretched hand with flexion or hyperextension of the elbow, leading to dislocation of both the radius and ulna.

2. Anterior Dislocations: Far less common, often caused by a direct impact on the dorsal side of the elbow, and may be further categorized into anteromedial or anterolateral dislocations.

Occasionally, isolated dislocations of the radius or ulna may occur. A notable example includes the Monteggia fracture—characterized by a radioulnar dislocation coupled with a fracture of the proximal third of the ulnar shaft. Another rare injury is the "terrible triad" of the elbow: a combination of elbow dislocation, radial head or neck fracture, and coronoid fracture. This underscores the importance of investigating potential concurrent fractures in seemingly isolated dislocations.

Clinical Evaluation

History and Physical Examination

Patients often present with the arm flexed at about a 45-degree angle, accompanied by swelling, tenderness, and joint deformity. Key physical indicators include abnormal alignment in the three-point anatomical triangle (olecranon, medial, and lateral epicondyles), strongly indicative of dislocation.

Neurovascular compromise, notably involving the ulnar nerve, occurs in 10% to 15% of cases, though median and radial nerves or the brachial artery can also be impacted. Differentiating dislocations from complex distal humerus fractures may be challenging in cases with extensive elbow swelling.

Diagnostic Imaging

Anteroposterior (AP) and lateral radiographic views are essential to evaluate associated fractures in structures like the coronoid process, radial head, capitellum, and olecranon. Computed tomography (CT) may be warranted for detailed assessment, particularly for preoperative planning in complex cases. Additionally, duplex Doppler ultrasound can facilitate early detection of brachial artery injuries.

Management Approach

Reduction Techniques

A straightforward elbow dislocation can often be reduced using a closed technique, involving adequate sedation, and application of gentle traction and countertraction. Occasionally, medial or postero-lateral dislocations require lateral adjustments during the reduction. Since a stable elbow joint dislocation may lead to substantial soft tissue damage and instability, monitoring for compartment syndrome post-reduction is crucial.

To assess joint stability, various tests such as valgus, varus, and lateral pivot-shift tests are used. A smooth joint movement post-reduction is expected; resistance or crepitation during the mid-range could suggest an incongruent reduction or soft tissue entrapment, often associated with coronoid process or epicondylar fractures. Any remaining flexion or extension limitations may indicate a loose bone fragment or a capsular tear.

Post-Reduction Care

Following successful reduction, radiographs should confirm both joint relocation and fracture status. The joint is then immobilized at 90 degrees of flexion in a posterior splint, avoiding cylinder casts to reduce the risk of severe soft tissue swelling. Current research suggests that early mobilization, compared to plaster immobilization, results in improved range of motion, reduced pain, and better functional outcomes, as prolonged immobilization can cause joint stiffness.

Surgical Considerations

Generally, surgical intervention is reserved for cases with concurrent fractures, persistent joint instability, or neurovascular injuries. Evidence shows minimal difference in outcomes between surgical ligament repair and conservative immobilization in simple dislocations. Irreducible dislocations, those with neurovascular complications, and cases involving open fractures or dislocations necessitate orthopedic intervention.

Ulnar Nerve Injuries

Ulnar nerve injuries occur in approximately 10% to 15% of elbow dislocations, with most cases being neuropraxic and manageable conservatively. Persistent numbness in the little finger is a sensitive indicator of ulnar nerve involvement.

Disposition and Follow-Up

Most patients with stable joints post-reduction can be discharged from the emergency department with a pressure bandage and advised on analgesia. For unstable dislocations, plaster immobilization and a broad arm sling are recommended. Follow-up care includes arranging early mobilization within two weeks to ensure optimal functional recovery without raising the risk of instability or recurrence.

Chapter 9 (C)
Fractures of the Proximal Humerus

Introduction

The functionality of the upper limb relies heavily on an intact shoulder girdle, which in turn depends on the proper condition of muscles, tendons, ligaments, bones, joints, blood vessels, and nerves. Humerus fractures significantly impair the effectiveness of upper limb function and are categorized into three segments: proximal (above the surgical neck), middle (shaft), and distal (supracondylar).

Fractures of the Proximal Humerus

Injury Patterns Proximal humerus fractures account for 5% of all fractures seen in emergency departments and

25% of humerus fractures. These fractures are most often seen in elderly, osteoporotic women, typically resulting from a fall on an outstretched arm. While most cases do not require surgery and can be managed in the emergency department, some fractures, particularly those with non-viable humeral heads, need early surgical intervention. Additionally, humerus fractures may occur in patients with multiple injuries or elderly individuals with concurrent femoral neck fractures.

Clinical Assessment Following injury, patients often present holding the injured arm close to the body, with complaints of pain, swelling, and tenderness in the shoulder and upper arm. Bruising may appear days after the injury, tracking down the arm due to gravity. Neurovascular examination is critical as the axillary nerve, brachial plexus, or axillary artery may be affected, especially with symptoms such as altered sensation in the deltoid insertion area or diminished muscle function. Given the prevalence of these injuries in elderly patients, it is essential to investigate any underlying medical conditions that may have contributed to the fall.

Diagnostic Imaging Three standard radiographic views—antero-posterior, lateral, and axillary—are typically sufficient to identify proximal humeral fractures.

Classification of Fractures Though most fractures can be managed conservatively in the ED, it is crucial to identify cases that need orthopedic intervention. The Neer classification system categorizes fractures based on the number and displacement of four anatomical areas: humeral head, shaft, greater tuberosity, and lesser tuberosity.

One-Part Fractures: Constituting 80% of proximal humeral fractures, these have fracture lines without significant displacement.

Two-Part Fractures: Representing 10% of cases,

these involve one displaced or angulated fragment.

Three- and Four-Part Fractures: Comprise the remaining 10%, with two or more significantly displaced or angulated fragments.

Treatment One- and two-part fractures are often managed with a sling and pain control, typically yielding a positive prognosis. For two-part fractures with displaced fragments, treatment options range from closed to open reduction, contingent on neurovascular status, rotator cuff condition, and the likelihood of fracture union. Open reduction and internal fixation (ORIF) are generally recommended for three- and four-part fractures, although recent studies suggest non-operative treatment may yield high rates of healing with fewer complications. Factors such as humeral head viability should guide surgical decisions, and newer locking-plate technologies may offer improved outcomes for unstable fractures.

Special Considerations

1. Fractures at the Anatomical Neck and Articular Surface: These fractures are rare but critical due to their risk of avascular necrosis, which may necessitate humeral hemiarthroplasty.

2. Fracture Dislocations: About 15% of anterior shoulder dislocations involve greater tuberosity fractures, sometimes with rotator cuff tears. Proper reduction typically aligns the fracture, although some cases require surgical repair.

Disposition Patients with non-displaced one- and two-part fractures are usually discharged with a sling, pain management, and instructions for early movement. High-risk cases, such as displaced fractures or those with other complicating factors, require orthopedic consultation and potentially hospital admission. Low-energy fractures, especially in older adults, suggest possible osteoporosis, warranting further evaluation with bone density tests and vitamin D assessments.

Fractures of the Humeral Shaft

Injury Patterns Humeral shaft fractures commonly occur in young men (third decade) and elderly osteoporotic women (seventh decade), with the mid-shaft representing 60% of such fractures. These fractures frequently lead to neurovascular injuries due to their proximity to the radial nerve and brachial artery. Blunt force injuries often produce transverse fractures, while falls with twisting forces result in spiral fractures. Pathological fractures, especially secondary to metastatic breast cancer, are also common.

Clinical Presentation Patients often support the injured forearm, with the elbow flexed and held against the chest. Common signs include tenderness, swelling, possible deformity, and skin tension or disruption near the fracture. Thorough assessment of adjacent joints (shoulder and elbow) is necessary to rule out associated fractures or dislocations.

Essential Management Points

1. Non-surgical Approach for One- and Two-Part Fractures: These can usually be managed with a sling and pain relief.

2. Surgical Options for Displaced Fractures: Options include open or closed reduction based on injury complexity and patient-specific factors, like neurovascular involvement and rotator cuff integrity.

3. Specialized Cases: For high-risk fractures and those involving anatomical neck dislocations, timely orthopedic assessment and surgical intervention are often required.

Assessment of the brachial artery and vein, along with the ulnar, median, and radial nerves, is essential in cases of humeral fractures. Radial nerve injury is the most common complication, occurring from the injury itself or as a result of fracture reduction. It manifests as wrist drop and sensory changes in the first dorsal web space. Studies indicate that radial nerve injury occurs in approximately 11% of mid-shaft humeral fractures.

Clinical Evaluation and Imaging

Radiographic assessment, typically using anteroposterior and lateral views, is crucial for accurate diagnosis.

Management and Treatment

Most humeral fractures are uncomplicated, closed fractures that can be managed conservatively with immobilization and pain relief. Immobilization options include a hanging cast, U-shaped cast, or functional bracing with a broad arm or collar-and-cuff sling. An acceptable deformity is up to 20 degrees of anteroposterior angulation and 30 degrees of varus-valgus angulation, with union rates exceeding 90%. Early specialist follow-up is advised.

Functional bracing is sometimes preferred over a U-shaped plaster, as it allows more functional use without compromising fracture alignment or healing. For oblique or spiral fractures, some orthopedic surgeons may recommend surgical intervention for enhanced functional outcomes.

Surgical repair is warranted for open fractures and cases with vascular compromise. Although radial nerve injuries commonly present as neuropraxia and often resolve without surgery, orthopedic evaluation for possible operative exploration is essential on a case-by-case basis.

Distal Humerus Fractures

Distal humerus fractures in adults are relatively rare and often follow the two-column anatomical structure of the humerus (the condyles). Classification systems, such as the AO/ASIF or Association for the Study of Internal Fixation, categorize these injuries into three types: Type A (extra-articular), Type B (partial articular), and Type C (complete articular). Practical classifications further divide them into supracondylar and intercondylar fractures. Supracondylar fractures are typically transverse, while intercondylar fractures may present in T or Y patterns due to vertical separation between the condyles.

Injury mechanisms often involve a direct impact to a flexed or extended elbow, causing the olecranon to drive upward, potentially leading to condylar fractures in a T or Y configuration or even fracturing off one condyle.

Clinical Assessment and Imaging

Patients with distal humerus fractures present with a swollen, tender, and deformed elbow. Skin disruption over the bone requires careful examination for potential compound fractures. Neurological and vascular assessments are vital, as nerve injury rates in these cases can be as high as 12–20%.

Radiographic evaluation should include anteroposterior and lateral views, though an internal oblique view may enhance diagnostic accuracy. Pain and restricted elbow extension may result in suboptimal radiographs. In cases of severe injury or soft tissue swelling, early CT scanning is recommended for more detailed assessment, particularly in intra-articular fractures.

If fractures are not visible on radiographs, the presence of a posterior or anterior fat pad sign may indicate an underlying hemarthrosis. Ultrasonography, CT, and MRI can further improve diagnostic accuracy and inform management, particularly for occult, intra-articular fractures.

Treatment and Management

For uncomplicated, undisplaced closed fractures with minimal swelling, immobilization in 90 degrees flexion using an above-elbow cast and a broad arm sling for three weeks is typically sufficient, followed by active mobilization. Cases with significant swelling, open fractures, displaced fractures, or neurovascular compromise require urgent orthopedic intervention.

Chapter 9 (D)
Radial Head Fractures: Comprehensive Clinical Overview

Clinical Presentation

History:

Radial head fractures are common, typically resulting from a fall on an outstretched hand or, less frequently, a direct lateral impact on the elbow. Patients usually present with elbow pain and restricted movement, particularly in forearm rotation and elbow extension.

Examination:

On examination, localized swelling and tenderness over the radial head are often noted. Subtle injuries may require forearm rotation with palpation of the radial head to elicit tenderness. Severe fractures may cause proximal displacement of the radius, potentially disrupting the interosseous membrane and causing distal radioulnar joint subluxation (Essex-Lopresti injury).

Diagnostic Investigations

Imaging:

Initial evaluation includes standard anteroposterior (AP) and lateral X-rays of the elbow, and sometimes the wrist if needed. A radio-capitellar view may help detect subtle fractures. The anterior fat pad sign on X-ray, often seen in about 50% of cases, suggests an underlying radial head or neck fracture. If pain or restricted movement persists, further imaging with repeat X-rays or a CT scan may be necessary.

Classification of Radial Head Fractures

Radial head fractures are typically categorized by the modified Mason classification:

Type I: Displacement <2 mm

Type II: Displacement >2 mm

Type III: Comminuted fracture

Type IV: Fracture with elbow dislocation

Management Approaches

Non-Operative Treatment:

Non-displaced Type I fractures and Type II fractures without a mechanical block are generally managed conservatively with a sling or bandage, promoting early mobilization. Short-term posterior splinting (not exceeding two days) may alleviate pain if severe.

Surgical Options:

For complex fractures (Types II and III), or when mechanical block is suspected, early orthopedic consultation is advised. Mechanical block assessment can be challenging due to pain; intra-articular bupivacaine may aid in evaluation. Surgical interventions include open reduction and internal fixation or excision of the radial head, sometimes with prosthesis placement.

Radial Neck Fractures:

Fractures with less than a 20-degree tilt can often be managed conservatively. Severe tilts may require reduction under local anesthesia, with manual repositioning. Open reduction is considered if closed reduction fails or if there is substantial displacement.

Essex-Lopresti Fractures:

Proximal radial fractures may involve interosseous membrane rupture and distal radioulnar joint dislocation. Wrist pain should raise suspicion, and lateral X-rays of the pronated wrist often show dorsal subluxation of the distal ulna.

Complications

Complications are generally uncommon, but neurovascular injuries and compartment syndrome can occur. Movement limitations may result from articular surface disruptions in the proximal radioulnar and radio-capitellar joints, though such complications are rare in minor fractures.

Essential Points for Emergency Management

1. Forearm fractures are frequent in emergency settings.

2. The limb's external appearance provides clues for assessing reduction necessity and success.

3. Median nerve function must be checked before and after distal radial fracture reductions.

4. Stable fractures may respond well to splinting or functional bracing, with early movement aiding recovery.

5. Orthopedic referral is warranted for fractures that are compound, unstable, intra-articular, or associated with neurovascular injury, as well as those failing ED reduction.

6. Displaced fractures of either the radius or ulna may accompany opposite bone dislocations (Monteggia and Galeazzi injuries), with a high risk of long-term impairment.

7. Persistent symptoms without visible fractures on X-ray suggest potential soft tissue or occult fractures, meriting further imaging (CT, MRI, or bone scintigraphy).

To address wrist fractures and dislocations effectively, several specific techniques and protocols are recommended based on the fracture type and extent of injury:

1. Colles Fracture: Initially, attempt manual reduction with traction applied in either extension or hyperextension. Once traction is achieved, volar tilt is corrected by applying pressure to the dorsum of the distal fragment. Radial alignment is then established by applying ulnar-directed pressure. Reduction is successful in most cases, though approximately two-thirds of these reductions may be lost within five weeks,

primarily during the immobilization phase. Cast immobilization is typically performed with the wrist positioned in 15° palmar flexion, 10°–15° ulnar deviation, and slight pronation, although evidence suggests alternative positions (e.g., dorsiflexion with mid-supination) may yield better outcomes. Functional bracing allowing limited wrist motion has also demonstrated positive results.

2. Smith Fracture: Occurs from a direct impact or fall onto the back of the hand or onto an outstretched hand in supination, resulting in a metaphyseal bending fracture with volar displacement (often referred to as a "reverse Colles"). Closed reduction focuses on restoring radial length and volar tilt, followed by immobilization in an above-elbow cast with the wrist in supination and dorsiflexion. Due to instability, most Smith fractures eventually require surgical intervention, and early orthopedic consultation is essential.

3. Barton Fracture: These fractures involve the distal radial rim and may be either dorsal or volar. Mechanisms of injury are similar to Colles and Smith fractures, with associated soft tissue damage and potential radiocarpal joint instability. Minimally displaced Barton fractures may be reduced and immobilized according to fracture type—wrist flexion for dorsal Barton and extension for volar Barton. However, due to instability, surgical management is often indicated, particularly for younger patients, and prompt orthopedic follow-up is critical.

4. Radial Styloid (Hutchinson or Chauffeur) Fracture: An intra-articular oblique fracture of the radial styloid is usually caused by a fall or direct blow, often leading to carpal instability and increased risk of arthritis. Non-displaced fractures are typically managed with cast immobilization for 4–6 weeks, while displaced fractures necessitate orthopedic referral for anatomical reduction and fixation.

5. Ulnar Styloid Fracture: These fractures arise from forced radial deviation, dorsiflexion, or rotational forces. Minor avulsion fractures do not significantly affect the distal radioulnar joint (DRUJ) stability, whereas fractures at the ulnar styloid base disrupt DRUJ stabilizing ligaments, leading to potential instability. Management typically involves casting with the wrist in mid-supination and ulnar deviation. Orthopedic assessment for DRUJ stability is advised.

6. Carpal Fractures and Dislocations: Predominantly affecting young males, these injuries are frequently localized to the proximal carpal row, particularly the scaphoid. Treatment strategies vary depending on fracture displacement and associated instability. Non-displaced fractures can be managed with casting, while displaced or comminuted fractures may require surgical intervention. Scaphoid fractures, which are the most common, often require additional imaging to ensure

accurate diagnosis, especially when initial x-rays are inconclusive. Advanced imaging modalities, such as MRI or CT, may be used for more definitive diagnosis.

7. Wrist Dislocations: High-energy trauma often results in dislocation, particularly affecting the scaphoid and lunate bones. Dislocations may present with dorsal displacement of the carpal bones or with a specific arrangement, such as in perilunate or trans-scaphoid perilunate dislocations. Imaging, including posteroanterior (PA) and lateral x-rays, is essential to confirm displacement and assess alignment. Prompt orthopedic evaluation is crucial, as reduction may be required to restore wrist stability.

In managing these injuries, the primary goals are to restore anatomical alignment, minimize functional impairment, and prevent long-term complications.

Introduction

Hand injuries are a frequent cause of visits to emergency departments (EDs), with common types including lacerations (~50%), fractures (~15%), sprains (~8%), and contusions (~8%)1. Males are more often affected than females. Due to the intricate structure and sensory role of the hand, injuries can significantly disrupt daily activities. Precise assessment and management are essential, as these injuries, beyond the initial physical impact, often carry occupational and psychological consequences. Even minor injuries, such as to the fingertip, can result in work absences, income loss, and concerns about long-term hand functionality and appearance. A thorough understanding of hand anatomy and typical injuries is crucial for accurate diagnosis and treatment2. In the ED, prompt identification of cases that need specialist intervention is as important as treating simple injuries.

Clinical Features

History A focused history of the injury mechanism is critical in assessing hand injuries. Key considerations include:

Timing of the injury.

Hand positioning at the time of injury.

Type of injury (sharp object or crush), as this determines likely damage to structures like nerves and tendons.

Presence of bleeding or numbness, which is essential in assessing possible nerve or vascular involvement.

Environmental factors, such as contamination with foreign objects like glass.

Recording hand dominance, occupation, and activities is essential for planning treatment. Verifying tetanus immunization status is also necessary.

Examination A thorough examination of the hand should be performed in a well-lit area, using additional lighting as necessary. Dressings may need to be softened if dried, with an initial moist dressing preferred at triage. Proper pressure and elevation can often control heavy bleeding.

For a comprehensive assessment, standardized examination procedures should be used. Analgesia should be provided before examination, as hand and finger injuries are typically painful. Local anesthetic can be applied around wounds or as a digital nerve block for a thorough assessment, excluding sensation testing, which must be done prior to anesthesia. For extensive anesthesia, a wrist block with a longer-acting anesthetic can be applied. Visual inspection, comparing both hands, may reveal swelling, bruising, wounds, deformities, or discoloration, which can indicate circulation issues.

Sensation is tested by light touch across the three main nerves in the hand. Each digit should be examined for digital nerve injuries, as specific nerves cover distinct areas: the median nerve supplies the thumb, index, middle, and half of the ring finger; the ulnar nerve covers the other half of the ring finger and the little finger; and the radial nerve supplies the radial side of the hand. If the patient cannot report sensation (e.g., due to age or unconsciousness), the presence of dry skin in the affected area may indicate nerve damage. Motor functions of each nerve are evaluated through specific resistance tests.

Palpation of the metacarpals and phalanges, along with testing ligamentous stability with valgus and varus stresses on finger joints, can reveal fractures or ligament injuries. Functional testing should assess tendon integrity by instructing the patient to perform specific movements. Some tendon injuries may be evident, but others, especially partial tears, may not be.

Clinical Investigations Most information is gathered through history and examination, with radiographs required if there's bone or joint tenderness or deformity. Pre-reduction x-rays are necessary in dislocations to detect any associated soft tissue injury. X-rays can also reveal radiopaque materials like glass. Ultrasound, useful in detecting organic foreign bodies or infections, can also evaluate tendon integrity. MRI, though less readily available for acute cases, may be helpful in cases where soft tissue assessment is crucial.

Appropriate pain management should be provided promptly, and rings should be removed to prevent circulation issues due to swelling. Tap water irrigation is cost-effective and does not increase infection risk3. Simple wounds may be managed with local anesthesia and fine sutures. Wounds in low-tension skin areas may heal well with conservative management4. Digital nerve blocks are useful for finger injuries, applying anesthetic near the digital nerve at the base of the finger. A long-acting anesthetic may be selected for extended pain relief in crush or bone injuries. Studies support using adrenaline with lignocaine to prolong anesthetic duration safely 5,6.

Hand injuries can be dressed with a crepe bandage for compression. Buddy strapping may provide stability to stable finger injuries, and elevation helps reduce swelling. Minor injuries can be treated in the ED, while severe cases often need surgical referral.

Fingertip Injuries Fingertips, with their rich blood supply, typically heal well with conservative wound care. Injuries involving the terminal phalanx may require surgical consultation. Less extensive injuries (e.g., <50% nail involvement and no bone exposure) can be managed conservatively. Tuft fractures are generally stable and need only dressing or nail bed repair. Care involves haemostasis and non-adherent dressing. Complex injuries, such as large tissue loss, may necessitate skin grafts or advanced flaps, which trained surgeons should handle. Major amputations may require finger terminalization, which should be discussed with the patient to address function over finger length.

Chapter 9 (E)
Pelvic Injuries

Anatomy of the Pelvic Ring

The pelvic ring comprises two innominate bones and the sacrum. Each innominate bone is formed by the ilium, ischium, and pubis, joining at the pubic symphysis anteriorly and at the sacroiliac joints posteriorly. The outer surface of the innominate bone creates the acetabulum, a socket shaped by the ilium, ischium, and pubis.

The structural integrity of the pelvic ring is maintained by robust posterior sacroiliac, sacrotuberous, and sacrospinous ligaments. Injury to this ring can severely impact the protected neurovascular structures and soft tissues. When there is a break at one location in the ring, there is often an associated break at another.

Classification of Pelvic Fractures

Pelvic fractures can vary in nature, including open or closed types and being either stable or unstable based on the degree of structural compromise. These fractures may be linked to hemodynamic instability, damage to hollow organs, or neurological impairment.

Young and Resnik Classification

The Young and Resnik classification categorizes pelvic fractures by the mechanism and direction of the injuring force, excluding isolated fractures outside the bony ring and acetabular fractures.

Most pelvic fractures are caused by lateral compression, anteroposterior compression, or vertical shear forces, all suggested by the injury mechanism and confirmed through radiographic imaging.

Types of Compression Injuries

1. Lateral Compression Injuries

Accounting for approximately 50% of pelvic fractures, lateral compression injuries often occur when a person is struck from the side. These are generally stable fractures but carry a high risk of additional injuries due to the significant forces involved. Lateral compression injuries may involve fractures of the pubic ram and potential sacral impact. Type 1: The most common form, with a sacral compression injury and anterior fractures of the pubic rami. These fractures typically remain stable and are confined to one side.

Type 2: Caused by more severe compression, involving iliac wing fractures and partial sacroiliac joint disruption. Stability depends on the sacroiliac involvement.

Type 3: A result of intense lateral force that impacts one side while causing a secondary anteroposterior injury on the opposite side, resulting in significant instability.

2. Anteroposterior Compression Injuries

Making up about 25% of pelvic fractures, these injuries are caused by forces applied directly or indirectly from the front, resulting in "open-book" fractures.

Type 1: These involve minimal diastasis (<2.5 cm) at the pubic symphysis without major posterior damage, generally stable.

Type 2: A more severe "open-book" injury, with ligamentous tears and diastasis of more than 2.5 cm. These injuries require considerable force and are commonly unstable.

Type 3: Involve disruption of all pelvic ligaments on one side, leading to lateral displacement of the hemipelvis. These are highly unstable, with a significant risk of hemorrhage.

3. Vertical Shear Injuries (Malgaigne Fracture)

Representing around 5% of pelvic fractures, these injuries occur due to vertical forces, often seen in falls or vehicle collisions. The hemipelvis is displaced vertically, frequently leading to considerable blood loss and potential intra-abdominal injury.

Clinical Assessment of Pelvic Fractures

A standard trauma protocol is followed, emphasizing the primary assessment and stabilization of airway, breathing, and circulation

(ABCs). The abdomen, perineum, rectum, and vagina are examined for evidence of injury, including signs of blood or neurovascular impairment.

A pelvic examination is part of the trauma assessment, with the pelvic region inspected for bruising, abrasions, or deformities. The evaluation should be done carefully by experienced personnel to avoid disturbing any clotting that may have formed.

Radiographic Assessment

Initial imaging typically includes an anteroposterior (AP) pelvic x-ray to identify fractures or pubic diastasis. More complex posterior fractures may require additional imaging, often with CT scans for better detail.

Complications Associated with Pelvic Fractures

1. Hemorrhage

Hemorrhage is a severe complication, with potential bleeding from fracture sites or major vessels. Disruption of the internal iliac arteries or associated veins can result in life-threatening blood loss, with certain injuries (e.g., AP type 3 or vertical shear) more prone to severe bleeding.

Management involves immediate stabilization, often with a pelvic binder, and may extend to advanced procedures such as angiographic embolization, REBOA, or surgical intervention.

2. Genitourinary and Bladder Injuries

In about 16% of cases, pelvic fractures may damage the urinary tract, especially in men, who are at higher risk for urethral injury. Bladder rupture is usually associated with significant pelvic ring disruption. Imaging with a CT scan is recommended before more specialized urological imaging to avoid interference.

3. Urethral and Genital Injuries

Urethral rupture, particularly common in men with pelvic fractures, may present with blood at the meatus, perineal hematoma, and urinary retention. Retrograde urethrography is essential before catheterization in suspected cases. Women are less likely to suffer urethral injuries, but vaginal lacerations can occur and require thorough assessment.

Management of Unstable Pelvic Fractures

Management focuses on rapid identification, stabilization, and splinting in the emergency setting, with resuscitation and pain relief as needed. Unstable fractures demand a coordinated approach, often involving surgical intervention or advanced imaging for comprehensive assessment.

Open Pelvic Fractures

Open pelvic fractures are rare but carry a high risk, with mortality rates reaching 40-50%. These injuries disrupt the pelvic ring, eliminating its tamponade effect, which can lead to severe, potentially fatal bleeding and an increased risk of intra-abdominal injuries or subsequent sepsis.

Management

Hemorrhage control is the top priority in open pelvic injuries, and early surgical intervention is essential to minimize infection risk. Sterile gauze packing is used to apply direct pressure to the wound. Immediate repair of open injuries to the bowel and bladder, as well as debridement of bleeding wounds, is critical. Stabilizing the pelvic fracture is typically the final step in the treatment process. Despite advances in medical imaging and aggressive interventions, mortality rates remain significant.

Acetabular Fractures

Acetabular fractures represent about 20% of pelvic fractures and often result from posterior or lateral compression forces, making their classification complex.

Clinical Features

These fractures are caused by the direct impact of the femoral head, sometimes accompanied by hip dislocation, which may cause sciatic or femoral nerve damage, depending on the hip's position. A thorough neurovascular assessment is required. Acetabular fractures may also occur alongside other pelvic injuries, as well as knee and hip fractures or dislocations.

Management

While standard hip and pelvic X-rays may indicate the fracture, a CT scan is often required to visualize anterior and posterior fragments and assess ilioischial and iliopubic column involvement. Such fractures are typically referred for inpatient orthopedic management.

Stable Pelvic Fractures

1. Isolated Pubic Ramus Fracture

Common among the elderly following a fall, these fractures cause difficulty in weight-bearing and localized pain in the groin. For patients unable to bear weight with suspected hip fractures but normal hip X-rays, further examination for pubic ramus fractures is crucial. The FABER test, where the patient's foot is placed on the opposite knee to induce hip flexion, abduction, and external rotation, may provoke pain, aiding in diagnosis. Pelvic X-rays are used to confirm the diagnosis.

2. Iliac Wing Fracture (Duverney Fracture)

Resulting from direct lateral trauma, Duverney fractures cause severe pain during weight-bearing, a waddling gait, and tenderness or bruising at the injury site. Typically minimally displaced and rarely comminuted, they are usually evident on anteroposterior (AP) pelvic X-rays.

3. Isolated Avulsion Fractures

Avulsion fractures occur when acute stress affects muscle and ligament insertions on the pelvic bone, common in young adults during sports.

Anterior Superior Iliac Spine Fracture: Often caused by activities involving jumping, where the sartorius and tensor fascia lata muscles contract forcefully, leading to pain, tenderness, and swelling. Diagnosis is confirmed via AP pelvic X-ray. Treatment is generally conservative unless displacement is significant.

Anterior Inferior Iliac Spine Fracture: Sprinting or kicking can cause forceful hip extension, resulting in an avulsion fracture here. Pain is sharp and restricts active hip flexion. AP pelvic X-rays reveal distal displacement of the fragment. Treatment is usually conservative.

Ischial Tuberosity Fracture: This rare fracture occurs from strong hamstring contraction, often in younger individuals. Local palpation or straight-leg raising may reproduce pain. AP X-rays show minimal displacement. Conservative management is typical.

4. Coccygeal Fracture

More frequent in women, these fractures result from falls on the buttocks with flexed hips. Symptoms include pain, swelling, and bruising over the lower sacral area. If physical examination confirms the injury, X-rays are generally unnecessary.

Management of Isolated Stable Fractures

Conservative treatment, including oral analgesics and non-weight-bearing strategies, is standard for pubic ramus, iliac wing, and avulsion fractures. Gradual mobilization and physiotherapy promote recovery within 3-4 weeks, allowing patients to resume high-impact activities later. For coccygeal fractures, rest, analgesia, and stool softeners are recommended. A foam cushion can help alleviate pain when sitting.

Chapter 9 {F)
Hip Joint Fractures: A Detailed Overview

Anatomy of the Hip Joint

The hip joint, a large ball-and-socket structure, is formed by the acetabulum of the pelvis and the proximal femur. It is uniquely designed to provide both stability and a broad range of motion.

Blood Supply to the Hip

The blood supply to the femoral head and the inner femoral neck is primarily derived from the trochanteric arterial ring. This structure forms an anastomosis around the hip, with a small supplementary blood flow from the foveal branch of the obturator artery via the ligamentum teres. Branches known as retinacular arteries extend from this extracapsular arterial ring to supply the femoral neck and head in a retrograde manner. Intracapsular fractures, however, disrupt this distal-to-proximal blood flow, potentially leading to avascular necrosis (AVN) of the femoral head.

Avascular Necrosis (AVN)

AVN, or bone tissue death due to blood supply loss, can occur in the femoral head following hip injury. Radiographically, AVN is initially hard to detect but typically presents with increased bone density in the femoral head after about six months. Disruption of the trochanteric anastomosis in femoral neck fractures is a primary cause of AVN, which can also occur in cases of hip dislocation. Immediate reduction of dislocated hips is crucial; if done within six hours, the AVN risk is reduced to below 10%.

Classification of Hip Fractures

Hip fractures are broadly classified as either intracapsular or extracapsular. Intracapsular fractures involve the femoral head or neck, while extracapsular fractures include intertrochanteric, trochanteric, and subtrochanteric types. Incidence rises exponentially with age, especially among postmenopausal women due to osteoporosis.

Intracapsular Fractures: Femoral Head and Neck

Femoral head fractures are rare, often associated with dislocations and commonly occurring from motor vehicle accidents (MVAs). They are classified based on location and fragmentation. For instance, superior fractures are associated with anterior dislocation, while inferior fractures are related to posterior dislocation.

Management: Immediate orthopedic evaluation and reduction are essential to minimize AVN risk and improve recovery. Complications include AVN (15–20%), post-traumatic arthritis (40%), and, in rare cases, myositis (2%).

Garden Classification for Femoral Neck Fractures

Femoral neck fractures, particularly in the elderly, are often low-energy injuries. The Garden classification is widely used to describe these fractures:

Garden I: Incomplete and stable fractures.

Garden II: Complete but undisplaced fractures, inherently unstable and requiring fixation.

Garden III: Partially displaced fractures.

Garden IV: Completely displaced fractures with misalignment.

Management: Non-displaced fractures (Garden I and II) are sometimes treated conservatively, while displaced fractures (Garden III and IV) generally require surgical intervention to prevent complications like AVN and non-union.

Extracapsular Fractures: Intertrochanteric Femoral Fractures

Intertrochanteric fractures occur between the greater and lesser trochanters. In elderly patients, they often result from a fall, whereas in younger individuals, they are associated with high-impact trauma. Patients typically present with pain and an inability to bear weight, with clinical signs including limb shortening and external rotation.

Management: Early treatment is critical, as intertrochanteric fractures can cause significant blood loss (up to 1.5 L) and are commonly accompanied by dehydration and malnutrition. Open reduction and internal fixation (ORIF) are the preferred treatments, yielding better outcomes and lower mortality rates.

Complications of Hip Fractures

Mortality: Hip fractures have a 14–36% mortality rate within the first year, with increased risk in institutionalized patients and those with comorbidities.

Morbidity: The most common complication is AVN, even with optimal treatment, as well as risks of non-union, infection, and osteomyelitis.

Summary of Key Points

1. Hip fractures are a significant health concern, especially in the elderly, with

notable mortality and morbidity rates.

2. They are broadly categorized into intracapsular and extracapsular types, with varying management approaches and outcomes.

3. Prompt treatment is essential for hip dislocations to minimize AVN risk, particularly with posterior dislocations.

4. Comprehensive evaluation and management, including ORIF, are vital for intertrochanteric fractures, especially in elderly patients.

Allis Maneuver and Techniques for Hip Relocation

Various methods exist for hip relocation, many of which require significant physical effort. One commonly used technique is the Allis maneuver. In this approach, the patient is positioned supine with assistants on either side applying downward pressure to stabilize the pelvis at the anterior superior iliac spines. The practitioner provides longitudinal traction along the lower leg, keeping the hip slightly flexed in alignment with the femur and bending the knee to a 90-degree angle. Gentle internal and external rotation of the leg is performed to encourage the femoral head to re engage with the acetabulum. Additional lateral traction to the inner thigh may be helpful.

Other available techniques include the lateral traction-countertraction method and the Whistler technique.

Complications

The likelihood of avascular necrosis (AVN) increases proportionally with the duration of hip dislocation, particularly if reduction is delayed beyond six hours after injury. Approximately 15% of cases may experience sciatic nerve neuropraxia, which is typically resolved upon reduction. Persistent ischemic changes resulting in neurological impairment due to pressure necrosis occur in about 3% of cases, often affecting the peroneal nerve. Missed knee injuries, including patellar, tibial plateau, and posterior cruciate ligament injuries, are present in up to 15% of dislocations.

Anterior Hip Dislocation

Anterior hip dislocations comprise 10–15% of traumatic hip dislocations and are frequently associated with femoral neurovascular injury or unrecognized fractures within the hip joint. This type of dislocation typically results from a direct force applied to an abducted and externally rotated hip. When the hip is in abduction, the femoral neck or greater trochanter impacts the acetabulum's rim, causing the femoral head to be levered out of the socket, potentially rupturing the anterior hip capsule.

Classification

Anterior dislocations are categorized as either superior or inferior. Superior (Type I or iliac) dislocations occur when the hip is extended during injury, while inferior (Type II or obturator) dislocations occur when the hip is flexed. These types can be further subdivided based on whether they are simple dislocations or involve fractures of the femoral neck or acetabulum.

Clinical Assessment

Superior dislocations present with the affected limb extended, externally rotated, and slightly abducted. Inferior dislocations, in contrast, appear with the limb externally rotated, abducted, and flexed. The femoral head may be palpated near the anterior superior iliac spine in superior dislocations or in the obturator foramen in inferior cases.

A neurovascular examination is critical, especially in superior dislocations where injury to the femoral artery, vein, or nerve is more common. Hip and pelvic X-rays are essential to detect associated acetabular or femoral head fractures, and CT scans may be indicated if pain persists following reduction.

Management

A thorough assessment for concurrent life-threatening injuries is essential, as anterior hip dislocations often occur due to high-impact trauma. Orthopedic consultation is required due to the significant risk of vascular injury and the potential need for closed reduction under general anesthesia.

Complications

Early complications associated with superior dislocations include potential neurovascular compromise due to direct pressure on the femoral vessels. Long-term complications can involve post-traumatic arthritis and AVN. Recurrence of dislocation is possible if anterior capsular healing is incomplete, often due to insufficient immobilization post-reduction.

Chapter 9 (G)
Femoral Shaft Fractures: Mechanism, Classification, and Management

Mechanism of Injury

Femoral shaft fractures in adults typically require a substantial force to fracture the femur, especially in individuals without underlying conditions such as osteoporosis or metastatic bone disease. Common causes include high-energy trauma from motor vehicle collisions, falls from significant heights, or gunshot wounds.

Classification

There is no universally adopted classification system for femoral shaft fractures; however, describing the fracture's specific aids in assessing the extent of blood loss and urgency of treatment. These fractures can be classified as:

Open or Closed: Depending on whether there is a break in the skin.

Type and Location: Fractures may be transverse, oblique, spiral, or segmental, located in the proximal, midshaft, or distal third of the femur.

Fracture Characteristics: The degree of comminution, soft tissue involvement, and neurovascular status should also be noted.

Most cases in otherwise healthy adults present as transverse fractures, often resulting from direct force, whereas high-impact injuries can lead to comminution.

Stress Fractures

Stress fractures of the femur occur from repetitive mechanical stresses, commonly observed in activities like marathon running or military training. Symptoms include localized pain in the groin, thigh, or knee, often undetectable on plain x-rays. MRI or bone scans are preferred for diagnosis. Treatment is usually conservative, given these fractures are rarely displaced.

Clinical Assessment

Diagnosis is generally apparent through physical examination. Key findings include a shortened and externally rotated thigh with the hip slightly abducted. Palpation elicits tenderness, and movement causes significant pain. Although rare, neurovascular injury assessment—checking distal pulses, capillary refill, and sensation—is essential to rule out complications.

Vascular Injury

Vascular injuries primarily involve the rupture of perforating branches of the profunda femoris artery, which forms a localized haematoma without distal vascular compromise in closed fractures. In contrast, open fractures or penetrating trauma may damage the femoral artery, leading to potential exsanguination or vascular compromise. Any sign of expanding haematoma or reduced distal pulses warrants Doppler imaging or arteriography for further investigation.

Associated Injuries

Femoral fractures are frequently accompanied by other injuries, including fractures of the pelvis, femoral head or neck, hip dislocations, and knee ligament injuries. Approximately half of closed femoral fractures also involve meniscus or collateral ligament damage in the knee, although acute assessment may be challenging. Blood loss can reach up to 1.2 liters in soft tissue surrounding the femur.

Management

Initial Priorities

In cases of concurrent major trauma (e.g., head, thoracic, or pelvic injuries), those injuries take precedence. However, early reduction of the femoral fracture is crucial for controlling hemorrhage. Treatment involves pain management, circulatory stabilization, and fracture reduction before radiographic evaluation if imaging is not immediately available.

chapter 9 (H)
analgesia

In the emergency department, pain management is critical. Intravenous opioid analgesia is commonly used, with doses adjusted for effect. A femoral nerve block is a valuable adjunct for pain relief prior to reduction and splinting.

Reduction and Splinting

Immediate fracture reduction and splinting reduce mortality, control pain, limit blood loss, and decrease the risk of fat embolism. With adequate analgesia, fractures are realigned using longitudinal traction with the knee extended. Specialized splints, such as the Donway or Hare traction splint, are commonly utilized for temporary stabilization until definitive treatment.

Fluid Resuscitation

Significant blood loss (an estimated 1,200 mL for a closed femoral fracture) can lead to hemorrhagic shock. Prompt fluid resuscitation with intravenous fluids and blood products is essential. Patients are kept fasted, and an indwelling catheter is often used to monitor fluid balance and provide comfort.

Orthopedic Intervention

For adults, early surgical fixation, typically through intramedullary nailing, is recommended within 8 hours. Open fractures should undergo wound culture and imaging, followed by surgical dressing, debridement, and antibiotic prophylaxis (e.g., Cefazolin 2 g IV). Surgical fixation is scheduled as soon as clinically appropriate.

Complications

Immediate Complications

Early issues include fat embolism syndrome, hemorrhagic shock, and adult respiratory distress syndrome, particularly in comminuted fractures. These complications may emerge during the initial resuscitation phase.

Long-Term Complications

Delayed complications may involve non-union, limb shortening, and malalignment, potentially resulting in long-term disability. Early mobilization post-surgery is crucial to avoid complications related to prolonged immobilization.

In older patients (over 60), the complication rate for closed femoral fractures is notably high, reaching 54%, with associated mortality risks.

Detailed Overview of Knee Injuries

The knee is the body's largest and most complex joint, classified as a synovial and compound hinge joint, comprising both the patellofemoral and tibiofemoral joints. It allows for movement from approximately 10 degrees of extension to 140 degrees of flexion, and includes around 12 degrees of rotation. These movements are stabilized by ligaments categorized as either extracapsular or intracapsular.

The main extracapsular ligaments, the medial and lateral collateral ligaments (MCL and LCL), ensure lateral stability, especially during extension. Intracapsular ligaments, which include the anterior and posterior cruciate ligaments (ACL and PCL), maintain knee stability during flexion, with both ligaments being situated extrasynovial. Muscles further reinforce knee stability; the vastus medialis muscle stabilizes the patella, the patellar retinaculum strengthens the anterior knee, and the iliotibial tract reinforces stability in slight knee flexion.

Clinical Examination

Effective diagnosis of knee injuries begins with a comprehensive history, which should detail the mechanism of injury, force involved, swelling onset, and immediate post-injury weight-bearing capacity. Knee trauma may result from either direct impact or rotational forces and can include valgus (outward angulation), varus (inward angulation), or twisting movements. Immediate joint swelling, known as hemarthrosis, typically signals a cruciate ligament tear, bony injury within the joint, or dislocation. Swelling developing hours or days later, often from a serous effusion, may indicate chondral or meniscal injury.

Physical Examination of the Knee

A thorough physical examination requires the patient to lie supine. It is essential to assess both legs to establish a baseline. Initial inspection may reveal swelling, bruising, deformities, and signs of past surgery. Palpation should start away from the injury site to identify warmth, muscle condition, and neurovascular health, then move toward specific points, including quadriceps and patellar tendons, collateral ligaments, joint lines, and other bony structures. Active and passive knee movements should be tested for flexion, extension, and rotation, while the ability to lift a straight leg assesses potential extensor mechanism injuries.

Stability Tests

1. Anterior and Posterior Drawer Tests: These evaluate the ACL and PCL stability. With the patient supine, the knee is flexed at 90 degrees while the examiner attempts to move the tibia forward (anterior drawer) or backward (posterior drawer) on the femoral condyles. Positive findings may indicate ACL or PCL ruptures, with anterior drawer tests showing limited accuracy (56%) for ACL injuries, while posterior tibial displacement over 5 mm suggests a PCL tear (specificity 85%).

2. Lachman Test: More sensitive for ACL integrity, this test involves supporting the femur with the knee flexed 20-30 degrees and drawing the tibia forward. A positive result, showing greater tibial displacement compared to the unaffected leg, has a sensitivity of 86% and specificity of 91%.

3. Collateral Ligament Test: Applying varus or valgus stress at 30 degrees of knee flexion can isolate pain or excessive joint movement, indicating collateral ligament damage.

4. McMurray and Apley Tests: These assess meniscal injuries. In McMurray's test, passive knee flexion and rotation detect lateral or medial meniscal tears through palpable crepitus or pain. The Apley test, with the patient prone, assesses meniscal damage through tibial rotation with downward pressure on the heel.

Radiographic and Imaging Studies

Clinical guidelines for knee imaging, such as the Ottawa knee rule, help determine when x-rays are necessary, primarily for acute injuries in adults with specific conditions (e.g., age above 55, isolated patella tenderness, inability to bear weight). Standard x-rays include anteroposterior (AP) and lateral views, which assess joint integrity, bone structure, and effusions. Specialized views (oblique, tunnel, and skyline) assist in diagnosing specific fractures, including tibial plateau fractures or subtle patellar fractures.

Advanced Imaging

CT scans are valuable for identifying complex fractures, while MRI is typically reserved for evaluating intricate soft-tissue injuries or if an arthroscopic examination is not preferred.

Types of Fractures

1. Distal Femur Fractures: Often resulting from high-energy trauma, these fractures include supracondylar, intercondylar, and isolated condylar types. Distal femur fractures may cause significant pain, deformity, and hemarthrosis. X-rays provide information on the fracture's nature and displacement, and management usually involves adequate analgesia, splinting, and possible surgical intervention for displaced fractures.

2. Tibial Plateau Fractures: Representing around 1% of skeletal fractures, these are most common in elderly

individuals or athletes, often resulting from a valgus or varus force on the knee. Schatzker's classification categorizes these fractures by location and severity, with types 1 to 3 affecting the lateral plateau and types 4 to 6 involving both plateaus. Avulsion fractures, such as Segond fractures, suggest ACL disruptions and are markers for ligamentous instability.

Clinical Recommendations

Key management points for knee injuries include:

Immediate effusion should prompt further imaging to rule out significant internal injuries.

Initial physical exams might be limited by swelling and pain, so reassessment after a few days is recommended.

Urgent reduction and vascular assessment are necessary in cases of knee dislocation to prevent complications like popliteal artery injury.

A powerful contraction of the quadriceps muscle at its proximal attachment, coupled with strong insertion at the distal patellar tendon, can exceed the intrinsic strength of the patella, leading to a transverse fracture. These types of fractures, commonly involving the central and lower portions of the patella, constitute up to 80% of all patellar fractures.

Clinical Assessment

Examination typically shows pain, swelling, and bruising over the patella. The ability to walk and actively extend the knee varies depending on fracture type, an important consideration for potential surgical repair. Testing for straight leg raise in a supine position can help confirm the integrity of the knee's extensor mechanism. Patients with non-displaced fractures may still be ambulatory and able to demonstrate active knee extension against gravity, whereas those with displaced fractures are usually unable to extend the knee actively.

Radiological Evaluation

X-rays, including skyline views, are used to diagnose patellar fractures. It's crucial to differentiate a fracture from a bipartite patella—a condition where patellar ossification centers fail to fuse, affecting 1-6% of the population. In bipartite patella, the fragments have smooth, well-defined borders with minimal separation. X-raying the opposite patella may help in uncertain cases.

Management

For minimally displaced fractures, conservative management with full extension is recommended initially, with gradual increase in flexion after 2-3 weeks. Displaced fractures with over 3 mm of separation or 2 mm of step-off, and cases with inability to perform a straight leg raise, generally require surgical intervention.

Dislocations around the Knee Joint

Knee Dislocation

Knee dislocations, although uncommon, are typically seen in young males and considered orthopedic emergencies due to potential vascular damage requiring urgent reduction. Most knee dislocations involve tibiofemoral displacement, often associated with high-velocity trauma, such as motorcycle accidents. They are usually classified by the position of the tibia in relation to the femur, with anterior dislocations being the most prevalent.

Clinical Assessment

Due to frequent spontaneous reduction before hospital presentation, thorough assessment is crucial. Knee dislocations often present with gross deformity and can involve neurovascular injuries, particularly affecting the peroneal artery (20-80%) and popliteal nerve. Neurovascular evaluation is critical, as vascular compromise may occur even with normal distal pulses. Peroneal nerve injury can cause foot drop and sensory deficits on the foot's dorsum and lateral aspect.

Radiology and Management

Immediate X-rays confirm dislocation but should not delay analgesia and reduction. Early orthopedic and vascular consultation is essential.

Reduction under procedural sedation is recommended, followed by neurovascular assessment documentation. Delays in reduction beyond six hours increase risks of compartment syndrome and potential amputation. Angiography, traditionally standard for knee dislocations, is now selectively used based on abnormal pulse findings or ankle-brachial index below 0.9.

Patellar Dislocation

Patellar dislocations, often lateral, commonly arise from non-contact twisting injuries in the presence of patellofemoral malalignment. Lateral dislocations occur with the knee extended and foot externally rotated, with possible direct trauma to the patella.

Clinical Assessment

Symptoms include sudden knee instability, immediate pain, and swelling, with inability to bear weight or extend the knee. In spontaneously reduced injuries, a lateral force applied on the medial patella border (apprehension test) may help diagnose. X-rays are used to exclude osteochondral fractures, although reduction can proceed immediately in clear or recurrent cases.

Management

Reduction involves applying anteromedial pressure on the patella with knee extension, followed by immobilization for 3-6 weeks to allow medial retinaculum healing. Up to 50% of patients may experience knee instability post-dislocation, and recurrent dislocations may require surgical repair.

Proximal Tibiofibular Joint Dislocation

This rare dislocation, supported by ligaments and the popliteus muscle, usually occurs with relaxed LCL support during knee flexion. Commonly seen in athletic injuries, such as shot put, it may cause weight-bearing difficulty and point tenderness.

Radiology and Management

AP and lateral x-rays aid in diagnosis, with reduction under procedural sedation achieved by flexing the knee and applying counterpressure to the fibular head. Immobilization post-reduction remains debated; surgical intervention is rarely needed.

Soft Tissue Injuries of the Knee
Collateral Ligament Injuries

Injuries to the medial and lateral collateral ligaments, often sports-related, are classified into three grades based on ligamentous fiber disruption:

Grade 1: Ligament fibers stretched only

Grade 2: Partial tear, mild instability with firm endpoint on stress testing

Grade 3: Complete rupture with instability and no endpoint on stress testing

Medial Collateral Ligament (MCL)

The MCL, along with adjacent structures, resists valgus force and stabilizes the knee medially. MCL injuries, the most common isolated ligamentous knee injury, usually result from a direct lateral blow to the knee. Severe valgus forces may also disrupt the ACL. Saphenous nerve dysfunction should be evaluated, especially in grade 3 injuries.

Lateral Collateral Ligament (LCL)

The LCL stabilizes the knee laterally, resisting various forces when the knee is extended. Injuries often occur from medial blows to the knee, sometimes affecting the biceps femoris and peroneal nerve. LCL injuries are less common but can be more severe.

Clinical Assessment and Management

Tenderness, instability, and joint laxity should be assessed, especially with stress tests at 30 degrees of flexion to negate ACL effects. X-rays may reveal avulsion fractures in some cases, and MRI can help in complex cases. Conservative management is common, with knee immobilization, ice, and anti-inflammatory medications. Early quadriceps-strengthening exercises are essential, and surgical repair is considered within 48 hours for severe grade 3 injuries.

Cruciate Ligament Injuries

Anterior Cruciate Ligament (ACL)

The ACL prevents anterior tibial displacement and controls knee rotation. Injuries often occur in sports due to sudden pivoting with the foot planted. Less commonly, direct trauma causes injury through anterior tibial or posterior femoral displacement.

Clinical Assessment and Radiology

ACL injuries typically involve acute pain, swelling, and inability to bear weight. Anterior drawer and Lachman tests assess ACL integrity. X-rays generally appear normal but may show a lateral tibial avulsion in some cases.

Overview of Tibial and Fibular Anatomy

The tibia is the primary weight-bearing bone in the lower leg, connecting proximally with the femur and distally contributing to the stability of the ankle joint. Its triangular shaft, located near the skin on the anteromedial side, is vulnerable to injuries. The fibula, parallel to the tibia, has a head connected to its shaft by the neck and is palpable as the lateral malleolus distally. Both bones are connected by the superior and inferior tibiofibular joints and a dense interosseous membrane, with a distal syndesmosis that provides additional ankle stability.

Compartmental Anatomy of the Lower Leg

The lower leg is divided into four compartments, each containing muscles, nerves, and blood vessels with distinct functions:

Anterior Compartment: Contains the tibialis anterior, extensor longus, extensor longus, and peroneus , all responsible for ankle dorsiflexion. These muscles are innervated by the deep peroneal nerve, with the anterior tibial artery transitioning into the dorsalis pedis artery near the ankle.

Lateral Compartment: Houses the peroneus longus and brevis, which evert the foot. The superficial peroneal nerve supplies this compartment and provides sensation to the foot's dorsum.

Superficial Posterior Compartment: Contains the gastrocnemius, soleus, and plantaris muscles, which facilitate ankle plantarflexion, with the sural nerve supplying lateral foot sensation.

Deep Posterior Compartment: Includes the tibialis posterior, flexor longus, and flexor longus, which aid in foot and toe plantarflexion. The tibial nerve provides sensory innervation to the foot's sole, and the posterior tibial and peroneal arteries traverse this compartment.

Chapter 9 (I)
Tibial Shaft Fractures

Tibial shaft fractures are the most common long bone fractures and are often open due to the tibia's subcutaneous position. High-energy trauma, such as a direct blow, typically causes these fractures, often resulting in significant displacement, soft tissue damage, and possible fibular involvement. Compartment syndrome is a significant risk, with some fractures complicated by malunion or non-union.

Fractures caused by torsional forces often result in a spiral pattern, as seen in skiing accidents, and vary in severity based on the energy applied.

Classification and Clinical Assessment

Tibial fractures are categorized by:

Skin Integrity: Open or closed.

Location: Proximal, middle, or distal.

Type: Transverse, oblique, spiral, or comminuted.

Angulation and Displacement: Noted in degrees and direction, with details on rotation and fibular or joint involvement.

In clinical assessment, severe pain and inability to bear weight are common symptoms. Immediate neurovascular evaluation is essential, including capillary refill and pulse assessment, as well as checking for potential injuries to the ipsilateral femur, knee, foot, or pelvis.

Management and Compartment Syndrome

Immediate management involves pain relief, reduction of displaced fractures, and immobilization in a long leg cast. Compartment syndrome, potentially affecting 20% of closed injuries, may not be apparent immediately and can take up to 24 hours to develop. Increasing pain, diminished sensation, and eventual pulse loss indicate advancing compartment ischemia, often affecting the deep posterior compartment.

If clinical assessment is challenging, such as with an obtunded patient, compartment pressures are measured, with a pressure greater than 30 mmHg suggesting compartment syndrome.

Radiological Evaluation and Definitive Management

Radiographs (AP and lateral) of the lower leg are essential to confirm fracture patterns and detect associated injuries. Management may involve conservative treatment in cases without significant displacement, while operative options, such as intramedullary nailing or open reduction, are considered for more severe fractures. Intramedullary nailing has been associated with shorter recovery times and fewer complications.

Tibial Tubercle Fractures and Osgood-Schlatter Disease

Fractures of the tibial tubercle, common in adolescents due to sports-related trauma, are classified by Watson-Jones into three types based on the extent of displacement and joint involvement. Type I and II fractures with minimal displacement are managed conservatively, while Type III or more severe fractures may require surgical fixation.

Osgood-Schlatter disease, a differential diagnosis, results from chronic stress on the tibial tubercle. Unlike fractures, it lacks associated hemarthrosis and is self-limiting, with management focused on rest and NSAIDs.

Tibial Stress Fractures

Tibial stress fractures are frequent in athletes, particularly at the proximal or distal junctions of the tibia. These fractures are identified by localized tenderness, and while X-rays may be initially inconclusive, imaging later confirms the diagnosis. Treatment generally involves rest and gradual resumption of activity.

Ankle joint injuries

Anatomy Overview

The ankle joint is a hinge-type synovial joint that allows for articulation between the tibia, fibula, and talus. It supports mobility and stability, helping to absorb forces during walking and maintain balance on uneven surfaces.

Ankle joint stability is maintained through a combination of its bony structure, joint capsule, and ligaments. These structures form a ring centered on the talus, essential for stability. This "ring" includes the tibial plafond, medial malleolus, medial (deltoid) ligament, calcaneus, lateral ligaments, lateral malleolus, and syndesmotic ligaments. Disruption of multiple elements within this ring can lead to joint instability.

Key Points

1. Ankle injuries are common and vary from isolated injuries to severe trauma.

2. The Ottawa Ankle Rules are a highly effective tool for determining imaging needs.

3. Lateral malleolar fractures are the most prevalent.

4. Early mobilization is advised for ankle sprains.

5. Achilles tendon rupture is confirmed with the Thompson test.

Bony Mortise

The bony mortise of the ankle is created by the lateral malleolus of the distal fibula, the medial malleolus of the distal tibia, and the tibial plafond. This mortise constrains the talus, contributing to the ankle's intrinsic stability. The medial ligament (deltoid ligament) extends from the medial malleolus to attach at several sites, including the navicular tuberosity and the medial aspect of the talus. The lateral ligament comprises three main parts: the anterior and posterior talofibular ligaments and the calcaneofibular ligament.

Most ankle injuries result from excessive motion of the talus within the mortise, often causing ligamentous or bony disruptions that destabilize the ankle.

Clinical Assessment

Injuries near the ankle may include fractures of the ankle and adjacent tarsal bones, sprains, dislocations, and tendon ruptures. Evaluating a patient with an ankle injury involves a thorough history and physical examination.

History

Key information includes the patient's ability to bear weight, immediate post-injury swelling, injury mechanism, foot position at impact, and force direction, especially rotational. An inversion injury, for instance, should prompt an evaluation of the fifth metatarsal base to rule out avulsion fractures at the peroneus brevis insertion.

Examination

A full lower-leg examination begins with comparing the

injured side with the uninjured side. Note skin condition, bruising, swelling, or deformity. Palpate ligaments, bones, or tendons, beginning away from visible injury and including the entire tibia, fibula, fifth metatarsal, calcaneus, and Achilles tendon. Special attention is given to the malleoli, starting 6 cm above each malleolus and including the collateral ligament attachments. Palpation of the anterior plafond and talar dome areas in plantarflexion may reveal additional tenderness.

Assess the ankle's active and passive ranges of motion (inversion, eversion, dorsiflexion, and plantarflexion), noting any discrepancies that might indicate soft tissue injuries. Also evaluate motor and sensory function, capillary refill, and distal pulses.

Ligamentous Instability Testing Ligament instability tests, including the talar tilt test (for calcaneofibular ligament integrity) and anterior/posterior drawer tests (for the talofibular ligaments), should be performed only when fractures are unlikely. Analgesia is provided for patient comfort during these tests.

Radiologic Evaluation

For acute ankle injuries, standard radiographs (anteroposterior, lateral, and mortise views) are recommended, especially in cases of deformity. The Ottawa Ankle Rules (OAR) can help determine the need for imaging in less obvious cases, as they have a high sensitivity for detecting fractures in adults and children.

Ottawa Ankle Rules

An ankle radiograph is indicated if pain is present in the malleolar region along with any of the following:

Bone tenderness at the posterior or inferior tip of the lateral malleolus

Bone tenderness at the posterior or inferior tip of the medial malleolus

Inability to bear weight immediately after the injury and during initial assessment in the emergency department.

Additional foot radiographs may be indicated for specific injuries (see relevant sections on foot injuries).

Other Imaging Modalities

CT scans are useful for evaluating complex fractures, while MRI can be beneficial for diagnosing persistent ligament injuries.

Ankle Fracture Classification Systems

Several classification systems exist for categorizing ankle fractures, with the Weber system being the most widely used.

Weber Classification

The Weber classification system divides fractures based on the fibula fracture level, correlating fracture height with syndesmosis disruption and instability risk:

Type A: Distal fibular fractures below the tibial plafond level.

Type B: Oblique or spiral fractures at the syndesmosis level.

Type C: Fibular fractures above the syndesmosis level, generally indicating more severe instability.

The AO system further divides each Weber type to include variations in ankle stability.

Henderson or Pott Classification

This system categorizes fractures as follows:

Unimalleolar: Affects either the medial or lateral malleolus.

Bimalleolar: Involves both the medial and lateral malleoli, often unstable.

Trimalleolar: Involves the medial, lateral, and posterior tibial plafond regions, invariably unstable.

Management of Fractures

Non-Displaced Fractures

Nondisplaced bimalleolar Weber A fractures (<3 mm) with no talar shift are managed conservatively in a below-knee cast in neutral alignment. Orthopedic follow-up is necessary to monitor potential fracture displacement or need for surgery.

Displaced Fractures

Displaced fractures, including bimalleolar, trimalleolar, or unstable bimalleolar fractures, generally require orthopedic intervention. These cases are managed through open reduction and internal fixation (ORIF).

Special Fracture Types

Tibial Plafond (Pilon) Fractures: Typically result from high-impact trauma, often require surgical repair due to complex soft tissue involvement.

Maisonneuve Fractures: Involve a proximal fibula fracture and medial ligament disruption, associated with syndesmotic injury. Surgical intervention is usually necessary.

Ankle Dislocations

Ankle dislocations, often accompanied by fractures, occur from high-energy impacts. Most cases are posterior dislocations, requiring reduction and orthopedic assessment for potential surgical fixation.

Closed vs. Open Dislocations

Closed dislocations, though often lacking neurovascular damage, should be promptly reduced to minimize soft tissue injury. Open dislocations necessitate urgent reduction and splinting, with surgical intervention as needed.

Soft Tissue Injuries

Ligamentous Injuries

Lateral ligament sprains are the most common ankle injury, typically affecting the anterior talofibular ligament. Ligament injuries are graded based on fiber disruption severity.

Achilles Tendon Rupture

Diagnosed with the Thompson test, Achilles tendon ruptures require prompt diagnosis for timely management.

Chapter (J)
Foot Injuries

Anatomy

The foot consists of 28 bones and 57 articular surfaces, organized into three primary anatomical regions. The hindfoot includes the talus and calcaneus; the midfoot contains the navicular, cuboid, and cuneiform bones; and the forefoot is composed of the metatarsals and phalanges. The subtalar joint encompasses three articulations between the underside of the talus and the calcaneus, enabling inversion and eversion movements in the hindfoot. Midtarsal joints include the talonavicular and calcaneocuboid joints, which facilitate abduction and adduction of the forefoot. The five tarsometatarsal joints, known as the Lisfranc joint complex, form an arch between the midfoot and forefoot, providing stability to the structure of the foot.

Clinical Assessment

History

Foot injuries often result from direct or indirect trauma. Direct trauma can lead to significant swelling and fractures, while indirect trauma, typically from twisting motions, usually causes minor avulsion injuries. Key points to document include pain, swelling, loss of function, reduced sensation, deformity, and any associated ankle injury.

Examination

Begin the examination with the patient lying down, comparing both limbs for bruising, swelling, deformities, and skin abnormalities such as pallor or cyanosis. Palpate key structures, including the Achilles tendon, calcaneus, base of the fifth metatarsal, navicular bone, and the area beneath the second metatarsal head. Assess the patient's active foot movements, then follow up with gentle passive movements, comparing with the opposite foot. Subtalar motion can be tested by inverting and everting the heel, with a normal range of about 25 degrees. Midtarsal movement involves stabilizing the heel while pronating, supinating, adducting, and abducting the forefoot. Each metatarsophalangeal (MTP) and interphalangeal (IP) joint should also be tested for flexion and extension. If the pain's origin is unclear, ask the patient to stand and walk. Circulation assessment includes checking capillary refill, skin color, and palpating the dorsalis pedis and posterior tibial pulses. A neurological assessment covers motor and sensory function.

Radiology

Routine imaging includes anteroposterior (AP), lateral, and 45-degree internal oblique views. The lateral view provides visualization of the hindfoot and soft tissues, while the AP and oblique views focus on the midfoot and forefoot. For suspected hindfoot fractures, an axial calcaneal view may be requested to detect subtle calcaneal fractures.

Ottawa Ankle and Foot Rules

The Ottawa ankle and foot rules help determine the need for x-rays in suspected midfoot fractures. Patients with clear deformities require x-rays; however, in cases with less obvious findings, imaging is advised if there is midfoot pain and any of the following:

Bone tenderness over the navicular

Bone tenderness at the base of the fifth metatarsal

Inability to bear weight for at least four steps, both immediately post-injury and during the emergency evaluation.

These rules boast nearly 100% sensitivity and are expected to reduce unnecessary x-rays by 30% to 40%. They do not apply to suspected hindfoot or forefoot fractures.

Additional Imaging

Magnetic Resonance Imaging (MRI) may be warranted if a stress fracture is suspected, as it can detect fractures up to two to three weeks earlier than x-rays. Computed Tomography (CT) is particularly useful for detailed imaging of the calcaneus, subtalar joint, and Lisfranc joint, especially for complex injuries or when fractures are suspected but not evident on plain x-rays.

Hindfoot Injuries

Calcaneal Fractures

The calcaneus, the foot's largest bone, supports vertical weight and serves as a lever for movement, making it the most frequently fractured tarsal bone. These fractures often result from direct axial loading, such as falls from heights, and may be bilateral in approximately 7% of cases. Around 25% of cases present with concurrent lower extremity injuries, and 10% have associated vertebral compression fractures, necessitating evaluation of these areas as well.

Mechanism and Classification

Patients typically sustain calcaneal fractures from a fall that applies direct force to the heel. Roughly 75% of these fractures are intra-articular, involving the body or posterior facet. The remainder are extra-articular fractures, occurring in the anterior process, calcaneal tuberosity, or sustentaculum tali.

Bohler Angle

The Bohler angle, formed on a lateral x-ray by two lines through the calcaneus, typically ranges between 20 and 40 degrees. A decrease below 20 degrees suggests a compression fracture. CT imaging is often required for complex fractures and preoperative planning.

Management

Calcaneal fractures are known for poor outcomes, with up to 50% of patients experiencing chronic pain or functional limitations. Intra-articular, displaced, or comminuted fractures present a high risk of compartment syndrome and require hospitalization for elevation, CT imaging, and potential surgery. Surgery may be more suitable for younger patients or those with significant Bohler angle disruptions. Non-displaced extra-articular fractures typically respond to conservative management, such as immobilization in a non-weight-bearing cast for 10 to 12 weeks.

Talar Fractures

The talus supports body weight in standing and bears high loads relative to its surface area. Unlike most bones, it lacks muscular attachments and is stabilized by surrounding structures. Its blood supply is vulnerable to disruption, raising the risk of avascular necrosis (AVN) following fractures.

Mechanism and Classification

Talar fractures are the second most common type of tarsal fracture. Minor fractures result from low-impact injuries, while more significant fractures often stem from high-force impacts, such as car accidents or falls. Severe fractures typically involve dislocations in addition to the fracture.

Talar Neck Fractures

These are classified using the Hawkins system, with Type I being non-displaced and Type IV having the highest AVN risk. The risk of AVN increases with the fracture's severity and displacement.

Talar Dome Fractures

These fractures can be challenging to diagnose on standard x-rays but may show an ankle joint effusion. Specific talar x-ray views or a CT scan may be necessary for confirmation, as these fractures can lead to post-traumatic osteoarthritis if untreated.

Management of Lisfranc Injuries

Lisfranc injuries should be referred to an orthopedic specialist. Most cases are managed with closed reduction and fixation using screws or K-wires, followed by 12 weeks of non-weight-bearing activity. Despite prompt treatment, complications such as complex regional pain syndrome and degenerative arthritis are common.

Forefoot Fractures and Dislocations

Metatarsal Shaft Fractures

Metatarsal shaft fractures result from direct trauma or rotational forces to a fixed forefoot. These fractures typically cause pain and bruising over the plantar aspect of the foot, making weight-bearing difficult. There may also be associated Lisfranc injuries or phalangeal fractures. The second and third metatarsals, being relatively immobile, are especially susceptible to stress fractures, commonly seen in long-distance runners.

X-rays usually detect most fractures, revealing alignment, angulation, and displacement. However, occult stress fractures may only be visible on CT or MRI scans.

Management

Undisplaced fractures of the second to fourth metatarsals are managed with a stiff-soled shoe or walking boot, allowing weight-bearing as tolerated for 3 to 4 weeks. In cases involving multiple fractures, significant displacement (greater than 4 mm), or angulation exceeding 10 degrees in the sagittal plane, orthopedic consultation is required. Closed reduction and a non-weight-bearing cast for 6 weeks are often necessary.

Hallux (Great Toe) Metatarsal Fractures

Fractures of the great toe metatarsal necessitate more aggressive treatment due to the toe's load-bearing function. Non-displaced fractures are managed within 4 to 6 weeks in a walking boot, whereas displaced fractures generally require surgical intervention.

Metatarsal Head and Neck Fractures

These fractures typically result from direct trauma and are often multiple. Non-displaced fractures are treated with a walking cast for 4 to 6 weeks, while displaced fractures require orthopedic consultation and closed reduction to preserve the integrity of the transverse plantar arch.

Fractures of the Base of the Fifth Metatarsal

Fractures at the base of the fifth metatarsal are the most common metatarsal fractures, with two primary types. The most frequent is a fracture of the fifth metatarsal tuberosity, typically caused by inversion of a plantarflexed foot. This is an avulsion injury from the lateral band of the plantar aponeurosis and is transversely oriented. Rarely, the fracture extends into the cuboid-metatarsal articulation but does not involve the joint between the fourth and fifth metatarsals.

Jones Fracture

A second type of fracture, known as the Jones fracture, occurs at the metaphyseal-diaphyseal junction of the fifth metatarsal and is prone to non-union. It is commonly associated with activities like jumping or dancing. This fracture is distinct from the diaphyseal stress fracture, which occurs distally to the intermetatarsal joint in athletes subjected to repetitive microtrauma.

Patients with either type of fracture experience difficulty weight-bearing, and there is tenderness over the base of the fifth metatarsal. Passive inversion of the foot causes pain. In children, growth plates at the base of the fifth metatarsal should not be confused with acute fractures, as growth plates run longitudinally or obliquely, whereas fracture lines are typically transverse.

Management

Fractures of the fifth metatarsal tuberosity generally heal well with a stiff-soled shoe or controlled ankle motion (CAM) boot, allowing weight-bearing as tolerated. Non-displaced Jones fractures, where the fracture does not extend beyond the fourth/fifth intermetatarsal articulation, are treated with a non-weight-bearing cast for 6 to 8 weeks. For significantly displaced Jones fractures, surgical fixation may be necessary. Athletes may benefit from surgery, as it often results in a quicker return to sport.

Metatarsophalangeal (MTP) Joint Dislocations

The fifth MTP joint is most commonly involved, usually dislocated laterally when the little toe catches on an object. First MTP joint dislocations, though rare, typically result from hyperextension injury and usually present as dorsal dislocations. These dislocations are often easily identifiable, with the metatarsal head palpable on the plantar surface. Dislocations of other toes are more subtle.

Management

Most MTP joint dislocations are reduced using longitudinal traction under local anesthesia. Post-reduction, a buddy strap is used to immobilize the affected toes. First MTP joint dislocations may require open reduction if there is buttonholing of the joint capsule. After reduction, a plaster of Paris (POP) walking cast with a toe-plate extension is applied for 3 weeks.

Phalangeal Fractures and Dislocations

Phalangeal fractures are common, typically occurring from direct trauma, often to the proximal phalanx. These injuries cause pain, deformity, and difficulty walking.

Management

Non-displaced fractures of the phalanges heal well with a buddy strap, which reduces pain and prevents displacement. Gauze should be placed between the splinted toes to avoid skin maceration. Pain is expected for up to 3 weeks, until the fracture stabilizes with callus formation. Displaced fractures should be reduced with traction under digital nerve anesthesia, and operative fixation may be needed if the fracture is unstable, rotated, or involves the hallux.

Interphalangeal (IP) dislocations, although rare, usually involve the great toe and are reduced using longitudinal traction under digital nerve anesthesia. Following reduction, a toe-plated walking cast is applied for 3 weeks. Other IP dislocations are managed with a buddy strap once reduced.

Chapter 9 (K)
Osteomyelitis: A Comprehensive Overview

Introduction

Osteomyelitis is an inflammatory bone infection,

primarily caused by pyogenic organisms. While relatively uncommon, it is a critical condition encountered in emergency care.

Aetiology, Pathogenesis, and Pathology

Osteomyelitis predominantly affects children and the elderly. In children, the infection typically spreads through the bloodstream (haematogenous route) and often targets long bones. In adults, osteomyelitis is frequently associated with underlying conditions such as trauma, surgical interventions, vascular insufficiency, or diabetes, and commonly involves the spine, sternoclavicular joints, and sacroiliac joints. Osteomyelitis may also result from infections spreading from nearby structures.

In children, haematogenous spread often affects the long bones, while adults more commonly experience vertebral infections. Bacterial pathogens causing osteomyelitis are often specific to the patient's age group.

Pathology

The infection alters local bone conditions, leading to changes in pH and increased capillary permeability. This promotes oedema, cytokine release, tissue destruction, and the recruitment of leukocytes, which further decrease oxygen levels in the affected area. As the infection progresses, pressure builds up, leading to small vessel thrombosis and bone breakdown.

In severe cases, the infection extends into the medullary cavity, eventually reaching the cortical bone, periosteum, and surrounding soft tissues, forming an abscess. Chronic osteomyelitis is identified when sequestra (dead bone) form as a result of cortical bone necrosis. Occasionally, new bone formation (involucrum) develops around the infection site. In some cases, a sinus or cloaca may form as a passage for the infection to the surface.

Epidemiology

Acute osteomyelitis affects approximately 0.1% to 0.8% of otherwise healthy adults in the

United States, with an increasing prevalence of methicillin-resistant Staphylococcus aureus (MRSA) infections, particularly following surgeries. In resource-limited settings, infections such as tuberculosis and brucellosis are more prevalent due to agricultural accidents, poor wound care, and limited access to effective antimicrobial treatments.

Clinical Features

The hallmark symptoms of osteomyelitis are localized bone pain and fever. Patients may also present with a history of trauma or surgery, which serves as a possible source of the infection. In the pediatric population, symptoms may appear insidiously. In addition to pain, patients may exhibit swelling, warmth, and tenderness at the site of infection. Diabetic patients may present with a painless ulcer on the foot due to neuropathy.

Risk Factors

Key risk factors include recent surgery (especially joint replacement), trauma (e.g., puncture wounds), diabetes (particularly with foot ulcers), vascular disease, immunosuppression (due to chemotherapy or steroid use), intravenous drug use, sickle cell disease, and iatrogenic causes like the use of peripheral intravenous lines.

Examination

Patients with osteomyelitis may not appear overtly ill and often show few constitutional symptoms. Examination should focus on the site of pain for signs of swelling, warmth, and tenderness. In the elderly, localized tenderness over the spine may indicate vertebral osteomyelitis. Diabetic patients may present with a painless foot ulcer, while children may show malaise, irritability, and fatigue.

Investigations

Laboratory Tests: Laboratory tests such as white blood cell count, erythrocyte sedimentation rate (ESR), and C-reactive protein (CRP) may be helpful but are non-specific. ESR and CRP can be elevated in acute infection, but normal levels may be observed in chronic osteomyelitis. Blood cultures are essential, especially in cases of haematogenous spread, with positive results in over 50% of acute cases. Cultures from bone biopsy provide definitive diagnostic information. Chronic infections may involve polymicrobial organisms, including anaerobes, mycobacteria, and fungi.

Imaging Studies: Imaging modalities assist in diagnosis and evaluation of the extent of infection. X-rays may show periosteal elevation, bone resorption, or sequestra but are most useful after 10-14 days of infection. MRI is the most sensitive and specific imaging technique, particularly for detecting early bone changes and evaluating vertebral osteomyelitis. MRI also helps assess the spread of infection to adjacent tissues, such as the intervertebral discs and epidural space. In cases where MRI is contraindicated, CT scans can provide valuable imaging, particularly for long bones and spinal infections.

Differential Diagnosis

Conditions such as arthritis, bone tumors (e.g., Ewing sarcoma, osteoid osteoma), gout, and septic arthritis must be considered in the differential diagnosis. Septic arthritis may coexist with osteomyelitis in certain joints, particularly the hip and shoulder.

Management

Osteomyelitis management requires hospitalization, often involving multidisciplinary care, including orthopedic, infectious disease, and radiology consultations. Early surgical intervention is crucial for diagnosing the infection, obtaining microbial cultures, and removing necrotic tissue. Empiric antibiotic therapy is started based on the suspected pathogens, with staphylococcal infections being the most common. Vancomycin is used if MRSA is suspected. The choice of antibiotics should be adjusted according to microbiology results.

Prognosis is influenced by factors such as underlying conditions, predisposing factors, and the bone involved. Chronic osteomyelitis, particularly with sinus tracts, is difficult to control with antibiotics alone and often requires surgical intervention for eradication. In rare cases, squamous cell carcinoma may develop in a chronic sinus tract.

Prevention

Preventive measures include eliminating sources of infection, controlling infections before surgery, and performing prompt and effective debridement of wounds. Managing diabetic foot infections appropriately can reduce the risk of amputation, a potential complication of diabetic osteomyelitis.

Summary

Osteomyelitis is a serious bone infection that requires prompt diagnosis and treatment. Risk factors include trauma, surgery, diabetes, and immunosuppression. A combination of clinical features, imaging, and microbiological cultures is essential for diagnosis. Early intervention with appropriate antibiotics and surgical management is critical to prevent complications and ensure favorable outcomes.

References

1. Clement, B.D., Ammann, W., Taunton, J.E., et al. Exercise-related stress injuries to the femur. International Journal of Sports Medicine, 1993; 14:347–352.

2. Niva, M.H., Kiuru, M.J., Haataja, R., Pihlajamaki, H.K. Fatigue fractures of the femur. Journal of Bone and Joint Surgery - British Volume, 2005; 87:1385–1390.

3. Provost, R., Morris, J. Fatigue fracture of the femoral shaft. Journal of Bone and Joint Surgery, 1969; 51A:487–498.

4. Russell, R.H. Femoral fractures: A clinical study (abridged by Peltier, L.F.). Clinical Orthopedics, 1987; 224:4–11.

5. Taylor, M., Banerjee, B., Alpar, E. Injuries associated with fractures of the femoral shaft. Injury, 1994; 25:185–187.

6. Vanganess, C., DeCampos, J., Merritt, P. Meniscal injuries associated with femoral shaft fractures: An arthroscopic evaluation of incidence. Journal of Bone and Joint Surgery, 1993; 75:207–209.

7. West, H., Turkovich, G., Donnell, C. Immediate prediction of blood requirements in trauma victims. Southern Medical Journal, 1989; 82:186–189.

8. Scholten, R.J., Opstelten, W., van der Plas, C.G., et al. Accuracy of physical diagnostic tests for assessing ruptures of the anterior cruciate ligament: A meta-analysis. Journal of Family Practice, 2003; 52:689–694.

9. Bachmann, L.M., Haberzeth, S., Steurer, J., ter Riet, G. The accuracy of the Ottawa knee rule to rule out knee fractures: A systematic review. Annals of Internal Medicine, 2004; 140:121–124.

10. Markhardt, B.K., Gross, J.M., Monu, J.U. Schatzker classification of tibial plateau fractures: Use of CT and MRI imaging improves classification. Radiographics, 2009; 29:585–597.

11. Fenton, P., Porter, K. Tibial plateau fractures: A review. Journal of Trauma, 2011; 13:181–187.

12. Kendall, N.S., Hsu, S.Y., Chan, K.M. Fractures of the tibial spine in adults and children: A review of 31 cases. Journal of Bone and Joint Surgery - British Volume, 1992; 74(6):848–852.

13. Scolaro, J., Bernstein, J., Ahn, J. Patellar fractures.

Clinical Orthopaedics and Related Research, 2011; 469:1213–1215.

14. Nicandri, G.T., Dunbar, R.P., Wahl, C.J. Are evidence-based protocols for identifying vascular injury associated with knee dislocations underutilized? Knee Surgery, Sports Traumatology, Arthroscopy, 2010; 18:1005–1012.

15. Wijdicks, C.A., Griffith, C.J., Johansen, S., et al. Injuries to the medial collateral ligament and associated medial structures of the knee. Journal of Bone and Joint Surgery - American Volume, 2010; 92(5):1266–1280.

16. Linko, E., Harilainen, A., Malmivaara, A., Seitsalo, S. Surgical versus conservative interventions for anterior cruciate ligament ruptures in adults. Cochrane Database of

Systematic Reviews, 2005; 2:CD001356.

17. Muller, M.E., Nazarian, S., Koch, P. The AO Classification of Fractures. New York: Springer-Verlag; 1988.

18. Harris, I.A., Kadir, A., Donald, G. Continuous compartment pressure monitoring for tibia fractures: Does it influence outcome? Journal of Trauma, 2006; 60:1330–1335.

19. Littenberg, B., Weinstein, L., McCarren, M., et al. Closed fractures of the tibial shaft: A meta-analysis of three methods of treatment. Journal of Bone and Joint Surgery - American Volume, 1998; 80(2):174–183.

20. Wheeless, W. Wheeless' Textbook of Orthopaedics. 2018. Accessed from: www.wheelessonline.com. Accessed January 28, 2018.

21. Hooper, G.J., Keddell, R.G., Penny, I.D. Conservative management or closed nailing for tibial shaft fractures: A randomized prospective trial. Journal of Bone and Joint Surgery - British Volume, 1991; 73(1):83–85.

22. Frey, S., Hosalker, H., Cameron, B.D., et al. Tibial tuberosity fractures in adolescents. Journal of Child Orthopaedics, 2008; 2:469–474.

23. Balmat, P., Vichard, P., Pem, R. The treatment of avulsion fractures of the tibial tuberosity in adolescent athletes. Sports Medicine, 1990; 9:311–316.

24. Stiell, I.G., Greenberg, G.H., McKnight, R.D., et al. Decision rules for the use of radiography in acute ankle injury: Refinement and prospective validation. Journal of the American

Medical Association, 1993; 269:1127–1132.

25. Bachmann, L.M., Kolb, E., Koller, M.T., et al. Accuracy of Ottawa ankle rules to exclude fractures of the ankle and midfoot: A systematic review. BMJ, 2003; 326:417–423.

26. Libetta, C., Burke, D., Brennan, P., Yassa, J. Validation of the Ottawa ankle rules in children. Journal of Accident and Emergency Medicine, 1999; 16:342–344.

27. Plint, A.C., Bulloch, B., Osmond, M.H., et al. Validation of the Ottawa ankle rules in children with ankle injuries. Academic Emergency Medicine, 1999; 6:1005–1009.

28. Muller, M.E., Nazarian, S., Koch, P. The AO Classification of Fractures. New York: Springer-Verlag; 1988.

29. Martin, A.G. Weber B ankle fractures: An unnecessary fracture

clinic burden. Injury, 2004; 35:805–809.

30. Jones, M.H., Amendola, A.S. Acute treatment of inversion ankle sprains: Immobilization versus functional treatment. Clinical Orthopaedics and Related Research, 2007; 445:169–172.

31. Pijnenburg, A.C., Van Dijk, C.N., Bossuyt, P.M., Marti, R.K. Treatment of ruptures of the lateral ankle ligaments: A meta-analysis. Journal of Bone and Joint Surgery, 2000; 82(6):761–773.

32. Weatherall, J.M., Mroczek, K., Tejwani, N. Acute Achilles tendon ruptures. Orthopedics, 2010; 33:758–764.

33. Deng, S., Sun, Z., Zhang, C., et al. Surgical treatment versus conservative management of acute Achilles tendon rupture: A systematic review and meta-analysis of randomized controlled

trials. Journal of Foot and Ankle Surgery, 2017; 56(6):1236–1243.

34. Bachmann, L., Kolb, E., Koller, M.T., et al. Accuracy of Ottawa ankle rules to exclude fractures of the ankle and midfoot: Systematic review. BMJ, 2003; 326:417–423.

35. Judd, D.B., Kim, D.H. Foot fractures frequently misdiagnosed as ankle sprains. American Family Physician, 2002; 66:785–794.